AND THEY SAID IT WASN'T POSSIBLE

KAREN R. HURD

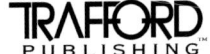

© Copyright 2006 Karen R. Hurd.
All rights reserved. No part of this publication may be reproduced, stored in a retrieval system, or transmitted, in any form or by any means, electronic, mechanical, photocopying, recording, or otherwise, without the written prior permission of the author.

Note for Librarians: A cataloguing record for this book is available from Library and Archives Canada at www.collectionscanada.ca/amicus/index-e.html
ISBN 1-4120-8212-9

Cover photography and design by Jonathan R. Hurd

Acknowledgements
Thank you to the following people who proofread the text: Gordon Waller, Ruth Hurd, Kathryn Hurd, Jonathan Hurd, and Jane Jeffries.

Printed in Victoria, BC, Canada. Printed on paper with minimum 30% recycled fibre.
Trafford's print shop runs on "green energy" from solar, wind and other environmentally-friendly power sources.

TRAFFORD
PUBLISHING

Offices in Canada, USA, Ireland and UK

Book sales for North America and international:
Trafford Publishing, 6E–2333 Government St.,
Victoria, BC V8T 4P4 CANADA
phone 250 383 6864 (toll-free 1 888 232 4444)
fax 250 383 6804; email to orders@trafford.com

Book sales in Europe:
Trafford Publishing (UK) Limited, 9 Park End Street, 2nd Floor
Oxford, UK OX1 1HH UNITED KINGDOM
phone 44 (0)1865 722 113 (local rate 0845 230 9601)
facsimile 44 (0)1865 722 868; info.uk@trafford.com

Order online at:
trafford.com/05-3178

10 9 8 7 6 5 4 3 2

To the Creator who made our bodies in such a marvelous fashion.

TABLE OF CONTENTS

    Foreword 7

    Preface 9

1 Rheumatoid Arthritis—The Raising of Its Ugly Head 11

2 The Twins—Ulcerative Colitis and Rheumatoid Arthritis 20

3 A Glimmer of Hope 26

4 The Nuts and Bolts of Ulcerative Colitis 30

5 Some New Thoughts about Rheumatoid Arthritis 41

6 Not Enough Grease 60

7 Sugar Really Can Cause Rheumatoid Arthritis 64

8 Other Little Nasties That Wear Out the Adrenals 81

9 The Little Nasty That Has Become a Big Nasty Because It Is So Misunderstood 91

10 Adrenal Helpers 98

11 The Lists 113

12 The Road to Recovery 121

13 What Could Be More Embarrassing? 128

14 It's a Good Thing I'm Home Schooled 140

15 Sometimes Life Is Like That 153

16 He's Just Not the Same Kid Anymore 160

17 Fingers That Stick and Feet That Burn 167

18 To Have More of a Social Life 173

19 But He's Just a Baby 179

20 Remove a Five-Year Old's Colon? 186

    Appendix 191

    References 194

FOREWORD

Karen Hurd's *And They Said It Wasn't Possible* presents a novel approach to the treatment of inflammatory bowel disease. She expertly lays out a pure dietary and lifestyle approach to controlling these diseases by using case studies to illustrate in layman's terms the logic behind her recommendations. Her explanations are well-reasoned, easy to follow, and enjoyable to read.

I have known Karen for over nine years and regularly refer patients from my family practice to her for nutritional counseling concerning a myriad of disorders. She routinely delivers sound, compassionate advice that yields positive results.

Karen truly has a servant's heart and her motivation for writing is to help as many people as possible. This book will give hope and help to thousands of families afflicted by inflammatory bowel disease. The results will speak for themselves.

Lane Woldum, M.D., Family Practice, Midelfort Clinic, Chippewa Falls, WI

PREFACE

The accounts that I have written in this book are true. Each client has reviewed their chapter(s) for accuracy. Some of the names and places may have been changed at the client's request for anonymity. The first account that I have written is very detailed with explanations and specific instructions of how to heal from gastro-intestinal disorders and rheumatoid arthritis (Chapters 1 through 12). The remaining chapters relate the stories of other clients without the specific explanations and details as that information has already been covered in the first account.

It is important to note that this work is not intended to discredit or demean the work of medical doctors. That profession is working as hard as I to help people get well. But, as I often say, there are many ways to skin a cat. Additionally, we have sometimes unintentionally made mountains out of mole hills. Know that there is hope. Know that your situation may not truly be impossible.

Karen R. Hurd, Nutritionist
P.O. Box 159, Fall Creek, Wisconsin 54742
715-877-3510, www.KarenHurd.com

1

CHAPTER 1

Rheumatoid Arthritis—The Raising of Its Ugly Head

Lyn reached behind her and rubbed the small of her back. It gave but little relief. The pain remained and continued to radiate all the way down her tail bone. Lyn sighed and turned her attention back to the computer screen. It had been weeks that she had been hurting, but she had determined that she was going to ignore the constant throbbing. She didn't have time for this type of thing. This project was due soon and if she didn't get it finished her boss would ...well, it just wouldn't be pretty.

It was almost nine p.m. when she finally pushed away from her desk, retrieved her coat, and walked out to the car. It was a good thing that not many people were left in the building because it was an effort not to limp. She managed to walk past her boss's office without showing any strain, but as soon as she knew he couldn't see her anymore, she gave into the pain. Somehow limping made it easier to walk.

Just getting into the car was difficult because she was so stiff. The burning in her tail bone felt like a small fire. She started the car and turned on the heat. The air blew out cold. She reached over and turned off the blower, realizing it would be another few minutes before the engine was warm enough to make heating the car worthwhile. As Lyn put the car into reverse and backed out of the parking space, she wondered how she had gotten to this point. Good grief, she felt like she was ninety years old when she was only twenty-nine!

As she drove home she wondered if stress had anything to do with all her stiffness and pain. After leaving Hewitt and taking this job with Abbott her stress levels had increased dramatically. She loved her job here and she thrived, in one sense. How could stress that she enjoyed make her feel bad?

She had risen to the challenge when she entered the male-dominated environment at Abbott. Everything was fast-paced and high demand. Something resonated within her when she was faced with a difficult situation and she was able to conquer it. She had been like this since she was a child.

Lyn's thoughts turned to the years that she spent in the Reserves—basic training, ROTC, Advanced Camp, and then finally making second lieutenant. There were times she had wanted to quit, times when she was embarrassed that she didn't understand the technical jargon, but she had persisted and won a commission anyway.

But there were some things that she hadn't conquered. Tears stung her eyes as she remembered the years that her mother had fought breast cancer. The up and down road of remission and then relapse had torn Lyn apart. Going through that with Mom had been so difficult. Lyn had felt so helpless. What could she do to change things? Nothing! Even now it grated. Lyn had always been able to change things. But she wasn't able to change cancer. The tears were flowing down her face now. Lyn wiped them away with the back of her hand. She had to get hold of herself. Mom had been gone for over two years. When would this pain stop? She had pain in her heart because of losing her; she had that blasted throbbing pain in her back. Pain, pain everywhere. Idiotic pain!

Lyn jammed on the brakes as the driver ahead of her decided to make a last minute right-hand turn. Stupid people! Didn't anyone know how to drive in this town? The anger of not being able to change the outcome of her mother's illness made her impatient. Lyn punched down on the accelerator, zooming by the tail end of the car that was making the turn in front of her. It wasn't long before she was home. As she turned off the engine, she realized she had been so upset that she had forgotten to turn on the heater. Oh, well, it didn't matter. She was home now. What did anything matter? She answered herself aloud as she slammed the door of the car, "Work matters. That's why I can't let this fool back of mine bother me."

Then Lyn suddenly realized—her back wasn't hurting anymore. Huh. That was funny. "Whatever, at least something good has happened," Lyn muttered as she marched into the house.

January rolled into February. The fast pace at Abbott continued. Lyn loved her job despite the huge amount of work that it entailed. She excelled in every way. Her bosses were very appreciative of her work; she received awards and raises in salary. She was truly happy. There was satisfaction in being recognized for what she did.

But it was stressful. Her whole life had been one big stress. At least now the stress was positive; she was seeing rewards for putting up with the constant strain. Lyn laughed aloud with the next thought. Maybe she was addicted to stress. Without further contemplation, Lyn focused on her work. The executive compensation package had to be finished by tomorrow afternoon. It seemed as if she still had a million phone calls to make before she could finalize the proposals.

* * * * * * *

Spring of 2003. Where had the time gone? She had been at Abbott for over two years. Lyn looked at her husband Jerry from across the small table where they were seated for a rare meal together. She had actually arrived home early enough to spend the evening with him. Not that she had time to cook a meal, but at least she had picked up pizza on the way home.

"Can you believe that we have been married for three and a half years?" Lyn asked as she took a bite of a pepperoni-laden piece. Jerry glanced up and acknowledged the statement with a shrug. His mouth was full.

Lyn turned wistful. "I wonder why we haven't been able to become pregnant. I want to have a baby so badly."

"Maybe it has to do with your stomach being in knots all the time. They say that stress has a lot to do with not being able to get pregnant." Jerry was sympathetic, but he also wasn't hesitant to point out what might be true.

"My stomach *is* in knots all the time. I even have knots in my chest. I'm always thinking, 'What have I missed, what might have happened, what might I have done wrong?'" Lyn sighed.

"Don't you see that you're worrying all the time? I know you love your job, but you fret about it incessantly."

"I do see, but I don't know how to change it." Lyn downed the rest of her soda and stood abruptly. "I think I'll go to bed early tonight. My tail bone is hurting again. It's probably all the blasted sitting I do at work."

The next morning Lyn felt no better. In fact, besides the pain in her lower back, there was something new. Her fingers were swollen and painful. Well, she had ignored her back for so long; she would ignore her fingers, too. She fumbled as she dressed herself, but managed.

It was a dreary spring day. Lyn glanced out of the window of the conference room. She was having a hard time focusing on the matters at hand. The pain in her back and hands—in fact everywhere—was so intense that it took considerable effort not to cry. She would not let anyone see how miserable she was! She plastered a pleasant expression on her face and concentrated on her co-workers' reports. She would conquer this somehow. She had to.

* * * * * * *

"You really should see a neurologist or something." Jerry hesitated before adding the rest. "You walk funny." Then he grabbed Lyn's hands, "And look, your hands are still swollen."

It was Saturday and they were seated in the food court at the mall. "I only walk funny because we've been tramping around all morning." Lyn couldn't stop the defensiveness in her tone.

"But it's not just today. You've been walking like that for several weeks."

Lyn didn't bother to argue. He was right. She knew it better than anyone else. Her hip stuck out to one side and everyone had begun to notice it, not just Jerry.

"Alright, I'll make an appointment with a chiropractor." It was almost a relief to agree. Maybe someone could help her.

* * * * * * *

Her appointment was not for another twenty minutes. Lyn had not been to this chiropractor before and was hoping desperately that she could help her. The pain was so intense today that the tears were slipping down her cheeks. Lyn left work earlier than she had to just so she could make it to this appointment on time. A thought struck her. Maybe the chiropractor would take her sooner! The pain was so excruciating she didn't know if she could wait until it was her turn. She stood up to cross to the receptionist's counter to ask if it was possible that the doctor take her early—but a popping in her hip froze her to the spot. Waves of nausea rolled over her as pain shot through her body. She didn't know that anything could hurt this badly.

The receptionist had her back turned, pulling a file from a cabinet. Lyn managed in a croaking voice, "Could the doctor see me early? I'm in a lot of pain."

The woman didn't even go check with the doctor. She simply said, "She's with another patient at the moment. It'll just be a few more minutes."

Lyn did not sit down. She didn't think she could. True to the receptionist's word, it was only a few more minutes until the door opened and her name was called, but Lyn felt like it was hours. Never in her life had she felt such pain as she felt now. Lyn shuffled into the small room that the receptionist showed her.

The chiropractor's gentle adjustment did bring some relief. Lyn wasn't sure what the chiropractor had done, but it had helped. By the time the adjustment was finished, the pain had receded into a dull ache instead of a raging fire. She was so grateful.

Before she left the room the chiropractor said in a calm voice, "You need to consider the possibility that you might have rheumatoid arthritis."

"What! Impossible. I'm not even thirty."

"Age doesn't seem to matter much anymore with arthritis. It used to be that only older people experienced the symptoms, but now younger and younger people are getting it."

"Humph." Lyn was not going to believe that. Obviously her hip was out of whack, that was all—otherwise the adjustment would not have helped. "Thanks, doc. Hopefully this will hold and I won't have to come back."

Lyn left the office and hurried to work. She had so much to do there. That report needed to be reworked and her boss expected to see the statistics on the new market analysis study. As Lyn sat at her desk a half hour later, a thought crossed the back of her mind as she immersed herself in the business of the day. What if the chiropractor was right? Lyn pushed the thought away abruptly. She had too much to do right now—she would have to deal with that later—if there was really anything to deal with.

The weekend came and Lyn finally decided to see if she could silence that niggling thought that the chiropractor had planted. After a few hours of research on the internet, Lyn pushed back in her chair and sighed. She was right and the chiropractor had been wrong. She didn't have rheumatoid arthritis. Everything she had read did not completely ring true. Okay, so she had a few of the symptoms of rheumatoid arthritis but the vast majority of the descriptions did not fit her at all. Her sigh was one of relief. She probably had just thrown her hip out somehow—why else did it stick out funny—and if she had to visit the chiropractor on a regular basis to keep her hip in line, so what? She could manage that.

* * * * * * *

Ah, summer in Wisconsin! Everything was jeweled green, the temperatures were moderate, and June promised to bring in a gently warm July and August. The stress at work had lessened somewhat and Lyn felt like singing. Maybe they would do some camping. Her heart was light as she went to bed that night.

But towards dawn Lyn stirred restlessly, wrapped in a fitful dream. Someone had her ankle in a vice. As the handle was turned, the vice clamped more tightly, and she begged her torturer to stop. A thought floating in another part of her sleeping mind told her that she needed to wake up from this nightmare. The grinding of the trash truck just outside her window had woven itself into her dream as a grinding sound in her ankle. Lyn's eyes popped opened and she jerked herself from the foggy tentacles that tried to drag her back into the nightmare. She had always grumbled about the early hour that the waste management company decided to make the rounds, but this morning she was grateful. The crunching sound of the trash being smashed had helped pull her out of the crazy dream.

Swinging her legs over the edge of the bed, Lyn stood up to begin the day. A gasp escaped her lips as hot fire vaulted through her ankle and up her leg. She fell back onto the bed.

"Jerry, turn on the light." The words were barely a squeak. Jerry rolled over and mumbled something unintelligible. Lyn reached out and grasped his shoulder.

"Jerry, something's wrong. I can't get over to the light switch. Please get up and turn on the light." Lyn's voice was edged with panic.

Jerry woke up and rolled out of the other side of the bed. He crossed the room and flicked on the switch. Lyn's eyes did not need to adjust to the bright light to see the red and swollen ankle that stared at her angrily.

Jerry was back at her side. "Good grief! Your ankle must be at least three times the size it should be." Lyn dissolved into tears. What was going on?

* * * * * * *

As Lyn waited in the white-walled little room punctuated with stainless steel accessories she went over and over the past few days. How could she have broken her foot, or twisted her ankle without knowing it? She had heard of people stepping off stools and causing hairline fractures that would create this type of pain and swelling, but she hadn't been on any stools. Maybe she had stepped down too hard on the stairs, or maybe ... The medical doctor interrupted her thoughts as he entered the room.

After a careful though painful examination, the doctor dismissed all her theories about a twisted or broken ankle. "There is nothing that is structurally wrong with your ankle. I think you have rheumatoid arthritis."

The knot in Lyn's stomach went from golf-ball size to basketball size. Lyn sputtered, "But I'm so young, how could that be?"

"We don't know why rheumatoid arthritis strikes. Our current theory is that it is an auto-immune disorder."

"What does that mean?" Lyn had occasionally heard the term before and read it frequently in her few hours of research, but she needed to know more.

"For some unknown reason the immune system attacks healthy tissue, causing inflammation and pain." The doctor's tones were reassuring as he continued. "I need to have some blood work done, and I'd like to recommend you to a specialist to have a confirmation in diagnosis, but if the outcome is truly rheumatoid arthritis there are many medications that we can use to help you."

Like a door being cracked open and letting sunlight into a dark room, Lyn saw hope. There were things that the docs could do to help her. Relief began to dissolve that knot in her gut. While she had the doctor's attention, she determined to bring up another issue.

"I need your advice in one more area. My husband and I have been married for a few years, and we would like to have children. So far we haven't been able to get pregnant. Can you recommend anything that could help us?"

"I'll give you a referral to an infertility specialist as well as to the rheumatologist. But you need to know that some of the medications that you may be prescribed for rheumatoid arthritis will not be advised if you are trying to become pregnant."

That crack in the door began to close. Lyn felt like she was slipping back over a cliff into darkness.

* * * * * * *

The specialist confirmed the diagnosis of rheumatoid arthritis. Lyn searched through the family health history and found that her great uncles on Dad's side had had arthritis and even the deformed hands. She couldn't have hands that didn't work! Her whole job revolved around using her hands on a computer keyboard. She couldn't go down this road! Fear began to eat away at her soul, and the tension in her life mounted.

"I have to function," Lyn told herself as she agreed to take the Celebrex that the rheumatologist prescribed. "But I still want to become pregnant." She firmly refused the stronger medications that the doctor recommended. She was doing her homework now. She spent hours on the computer researching arthritis medications and their side effects. She had become a mini-expert in rheumatoid arthritis. She would face this monster with increased knowledge.

She would do all that she could to keep from becoming deformed, yet still give herself the chance to have a baby.

The Celebrex helped the pain but did not alleviate it. She was able to function and do all of her work just as well as she always had, though she had to hide the tears that refused to be checked at times. Her boss knew about her doctor visits and the medication, but she would not let him know how much she really hurt. She loved this job—she needed this job. She could not let him see any weakness in her.

2

CHAPTER 2

The Twins—Ulcerative Colitis and Rheumatoid Arthritis

"What's this?" Lyn spoke the words aloud. No one was in the bathroom with her. She had come rapidly down the hall to the women's restroom as she always did when the urge to have a bowel movement came on her. That was nothing new. Ever since she was a little girl, when she needed to go, she needed to go *now*. But *this* was something new. She had never had blood in her stool. "It's only a little bit. I have too much to worry about right now. I'm *not* going to worry about this!" Lyn almost laughed aloud. Now she was talking to herself in the women's bathroom. What would Jerry say? He'd laugh, too.

But July turned into August and then September, and the bleeding did not stop. In fact, it grew worse. Now there wasn't a little blood in her stool, there was a lot of blood. No longer did she walk rapidly down the hall to make it to the ladies' room, she literally ran down the hall. And these urgent races were happening three to four times a day.

* * * * * * *

The exam was as much embarrassing as uncomfortable, but the general practitioner had to find out if it were simply hemorrhoids or if more investigation was needed. "There is no reason for your bleeding here. I'm referring you to a gastroenterologist."

"Great," Lyn thought wryly. She had a general practitioner, a rheumatologist, was thinking of seeing an infertility specialist, and now she was going to add to her already long list of health care providers, a gut doctor. Throw into the mix that September was the busiest month of the entire year at work. The hours were long and arduous, and the stress incredible. What could possibly go wrong next!?

* * * * * * *

Two days before the biggest project of the year was due, Lyn groaned as she woke up. The tears began immediately. Her knees were so swollen that she couldn't walk at all. She called her boss, unable to disguise her sobs as she told him the situation. His response was to get another drug, a stronger drug, so that she could function. Lyn could not bring herself to tell him that she had refused the stronger medications because she was trying to become pregnant.

Lyn wasn't able to go into work at all. She literally crawled to the kitchen table and sat there with her head in her hands. The pain was almost unbearable. *Why me? Why me, God?*

After a short while, Lyn managed to creep back to her bed where she spent most of the day on the telephone with the girl at work who was her back-up. It was the first time a co-worker had to cover one of Lyn's projects. As the day wore on, the pain lessened for some reason. It seemed the more absorbed she was in her work, the less pain she experienced. But the real trial came when she had to manage to get to the bathroom. *That* problem didn't lessen at all when she was focusing fully on her work. Bloody stools, searing hot pain that crippled her, inability to get pregnant! Why?

* * * * * * *

"Lyn, this isn't normal." Jerry was growing tired of Lyn's stubbornness. She continued to put off going to the doctor because of her busyness at work. "People shouldn't have to crawl down the hall to go to the bathroom." He grabbed her arm and lifted it for emphasis. "Neither is this normal." The red welts she had from simply scratching her arm would normally disappear within an hour but had been occurring for many days now.

"Okay, okay. I'll go back to the doctor." She *had* already been back again and again. Once she had even gone to the emergency room because the pain was so intense and the Celebrex wasn't touching it. But she had left before seeing a doctor because she had actually started to feel better while she had sat there like a nervous wreck waiting her turn. Sometimes she wondered why she felt less pain when she was agitated. It didn't make sense.

* * * * * * *

"I believe it's a reaction to the Celebrex," the M.D. said. He had thoroughly examined the large red wheals that looked like someone had taken a whip to her. "I'd like to try Vioxx instead." Lyn agreed. She hadn't read anything to make her believe that Vioxx was any worse than Celebrex as far as infertility was concerned.

Lyn religiously carried out the instructions of the doctor. She forced herself to walk at least fifteen to twenty minutes a day, four to five times a week. The doctor had said that walking was helpful in controlling the rheumatoid arthritis. The Van Patton Forest Preserve was her favorite place to accomplish this torture. But as the weeks passed, the pain mounted. In a moment of complete breakdown, Lyn decided to call the doctor on her cell phone while she was toiling through the Van Patton woods.

"Don't give me any of this 'he's not available' rigmarole. I need to speak to him immediately." Lyn knew she wasn't being patient with the receptionist, but right now she didn't care. She had had more than she could take. Amazingly, the doctor's voice came through on her cell phone in just a few minutes.

"This is not working," Lyn stated in a voice tight with pain. "I can't take it anymore."

The doctor's response was clear, framed in words that communicated his message empathically. "You're going to have to accept this, live with it, and take the stronger medications."

As Lyn snapped the lip closed on the cell phone, she felt like howling. "Live with it! Take stronger medications that would harm any baby in my womb if ever I was able to conceive one! No!"

How had she survived all this time? By sheer willpower. She *would* survive. She *would* somehow make it. Hard work had always paid off—somehow she would conquer this with or without the help of doctors. The powerful emotions of resolve and driving determination somehow made the pain she had been feeling just a minute ago fade into the background. As Lyn marched down the forest path, that mystery once again teased her mind.

* * * * * * *

Lyn's voice was firm. "I'll have to reschedule the colonoscopy. This project is due, and I can't afford to take the time to run off and do that." Jerry shrugged. Lyn was a strong-willed woman and he had learned to let her do things the way she wanted to do them. She managed a smile at her beloved husband, "And I'll be all right. Somehow, I'll be all right." Lyn wondered if she had said that more for herself than for Jerry. No time to ponder that thought. She needed to get to work.

The rheumatoid arthritis raged full force. It was probably the worst flare-up she had had. Lyn leaned on the Vioxx heavily. The project would be finished by the end of December. Then she would do the colonoscopy in January 2004. Wow. It would be 2004. Where did the time go? Then another thought—still no baby—and now they had been married five years.

By the time January fifth arrived, the day of Lyn's colonoscopy, the bowel problems had grown to such an extent that she was having eight to ten bloody stools per day. "I never thought I would be doing this," Lyn grumbled to herself as she packed up the extra pairs of underwear that she now carried with her to work. Between the incredible bowel urgency and the crippling pain of the arthritis, it was a too-often occurrence when she couldn't make it to the restroom on time.

It was just past noon when the urge hit her again. Lyn was in the restroom, the unrestrained hot tears making rivulets that coursed down her face. "I've never been a quitter, but maybe this time I will be defeated. I think I'm going to be forced to resign my position." January was one of the busiest months in executive compensation. She didn't know how much longer she would be able to continue to function like this. She was spending too much time in the bathroom when she should be working. Her boss hadn't said much, but there was no hiding the fact that she haunted the women's room like a gloaming ghost.

* * * * * * *

She was glad when the colonoscopy was over. She wondered if she had any shred of modesty left—between digital exams, infertility exams, and now colonoscopies—was there any part of her that was decently unexposed? At this point, she almost—just almost—didn't care. She felt like crumpling when the doctor gave her the results.

"Ulcerative colitis."

As the doctor explained, Lyn listened in shock. She felt like she was watching her life through a window—slightly distant and removed. The words "incurable" managed to come through as well as "medications that will only control the disease—you'll be on them for the rest of your life."

So began the regime of enemas every morning and every evening. But there was something that happened that made Lyn sit up and take notice as soon as she began the enemas. She had almost instantaneous relief from the rheumatoid arthritis. Calling her doctor she inquired about this wonderful phenomenon.

"I've read that the enemas are steroids. Do they reduce the inflammation in the other parts of the body as well as the bowel?" Lyn asked.

"No, I don't think so," the doctor replied. "Your rheumatoid arthritis is probably better because the ulcers have healed."

Lyn shrugged. That didn't sound right, but she let it drop. She had another question to ask before this call with the doctor was over.

"Will steroids harm a baby if I did become pregnant?"

The doctor's answer was vague. "We'll cross that bridge if we come to it."

Lyn didn't fight the doctor. It was too good to be true that she didn't have to rush to the bathroom as frequently, and the arthritic pain that wracked her body was practically gone.

Winter gave way to spring. All of the hope that Lyn had realized began to fade as she started to have difficulty in holding the morning enemas. She was expelling them almost immediately. She couldn't keep the medication in long enough to have any effect. The symptoms of ulcerative colitis and rheumatoid arthritis were back, beating on her door like a madman pounding for entrance. The doctor prescribed a suppository instead of the morning enema to facilitate getting the medication into her. It worked, but only for a little while.

Then the infertility testing came back negative. That was good news in a way. But Lyn felt like crying. Goodness, she was doing a lot of that in the last few years! It would have been better if they had found some problem that could be corrected. Her infertility was still unexplained and that made it all the more frustrating.

* * * * * * *

It was July 2004—barely seven months after her diagnosis of ulcerative colitis. Although her rheumatoid arthritis was in remission at the moment, the bowel trouble was getting worse. The enemas and suppositories were not working. Lyn was on the phone with the doctor again.

"It's a life-long disease. You'll just have to accept it." The doctor's voice left no room for argument, but Lyn was going to try anyway.

"Isn't there anything that nutrition can do?"

"There is nothing that shows nutrition can help."

"But isn't there someone you could refer me to …so that I could at least give it a shot? I can't live the rest of my life tied to a bathroom."

The doctor gave her the name of a nutritionist that worked in the same building. Lyn began to dial the number but then thought, "If the doctor doesn't believe that nutrition helps, why would I go to someone he refers me to?" Lyn put the phone back down.

That weekend Lyn decided to spend as many hours as necessary to learn all that she could about nutrition and ulcerative colitis. The internet provided a wealth of information and in her search she came across a web site that held her spellbound. There was a nutritionist out there that described Lyn's problems to a tee and had a solution spelled out. As Lyn read through the testimonies published on the site, one by a nurse caught her attention particularly. "This nutritionist knows more about the colon than anyone I know."

"Okay," Lyn spoke aloud to herself, "I'll try it. I have nothing to lose." Printing off a copy of the plan that the nutritionist had written, Lyn also e-mailed her to ask some questions.

CHAPTER 3

A Glimmer of Hope

Karen sat in her office. It was late. So many e-mails. So many hurting people. She sighed. "I need to help them." That sigh and thought had crossed her lips and mind innumerable times in the years that she had been practicing nutrition. Averaging a client load of eight to twelve people daily, she was able to keep up, except she did fall behind on her e-mails frequently. Again, the plans that she had been formulating to somehow expand her practice through the training of up-and-coming nutritionists came to her mind. Not yet. It wasn't time.

Here was an e-mail dated July twelfth. "Well, I'm only answering a week late," Karen thought, but she still winced. She wanted to be as responsive as possible. These people were desperate, disparaging, and without much hope. She knew how it felt to be in their position. My, how she knew! Her eyes rested on the little note that Ruth had written to her. "When my spirit grows faint within me, it is You who know my way." (The Bible, Psalm 142:3)

Her Ruth. Daughter snatched from the jaws of death. Every doctor had said the same: "There is nothing that can be done. Less than a few months and she'll be dead." But Ruth lived. By God's grace and the knowledge that he had given to Karen, she lived. That story was written in detail on her web site. That writing project was complete, for now.

Karen's eyes turned to the e-mail. She always made sure to read the entire text. These were people pouring out their troubles. They deserved her full attention.

Last June I was diagnosed with rheumatoid arthritis. In January, I was diagnosed with ulcerative colitis. Since January, I have been taking enemas/suppositories twice a day and my rheumatoid arthritis has gotten significantly better. I no longer have to take Vioxx on a daily basis. However, I get reoccurring ulcerative colitis flare-ups and do NOT want this to be a life-long disease. For goodness sakes, I'm only thirty! Tomorrow I begin the White Diet that you outlined on your web site, but I have a question, and I did not find the answer on the site. I get frequent headaches for which I take two ibuprofen. In addition, I take one Colocort enema in the evening and one Canasa suppository in the morning. Will taking these drugs affect the results of the White Diet?
Thanks in advance for your help.
Lyn Redmond, Bristol, Wisconsin

They need so much more than a simple e-mail response. They need to know the details. They need to know the "why." They need to know how in the world they got into this pickle and how in the world to get out. All of this passed through Karen's mind as she typed the response.

It is certainly possible that the ibuprofen, enema, and suppository could taint the results—but you should try anyway. If you need further assistance, feel free to contact me and we can set up a consultation so that I can help you with the problems that you have outlined. They are very easy to correct with diet alone.
Sincerely,
Karen R. Hurd
Nutritionist

Karen wanted to walk each person through healing. That way she would be able to deal with the curve balls that would most certainly fly. No health situation was cut and dried. Each person would have details to their situation that would not be clear in one e-mailing or one consultation. Again the thought came to her mind—"what will you do when you have so many clients that you don't have the time to walk each one through the healing process?" Karen answered herself aloud, "I'll cross that bridge when I come to it. Right now, I hope that this Lyn will contact me. She needs my help. And by God's grace, I think I can help her."

****

Karen had responded! Lyn breathed a silent "thank you." She had gotten home late, as usual. It was 10:50 p.m. on July twentieth. Lyn had looked for an e-mail from this woman every day. Finally, it was here. Jerry called from the other room, "Lyn, it's late. You better get to bed."

"I'm coming. I just need to answer this one e-mail."

Dear Karen,
    Thank you for your response. I'd really like to set up a consultation. I'm not sure the White Diet worked for me. Maybe I should have continued it longer than the initial three days? However, all it seemed to do was make me constipated with bloody "leakage" for lack of a better term. There's also a frequent urgency to go, but not as bad as in the past. Right now, I'm on Day 5 after completion of the White Diet—but, I have not taken any legumes today because I'm afraid they will make the bleeding and urgency worse.
    Please let me know the next steps for setting this up or do I need to go back on the web site to do this?
Thanks so much.
Lyn

* * * * * * *

Up late again. "A good thing that I work for myself," thought Karen. "I can choose to sleep in or take naps whenever I decide I want to schedule it." Karen glanced at the clock. July twentieth, 11:59 p.m., 2004. "Might as well call it July twenty-first. Just a few more e-mails and I'll be finished." She hit the send and receive button to make sure that was it for the evening. Three more junk e-mails appeared. Karen mumbled to herself, "I thought I had downloaded all the updates for the anti-spam program. Looks like somebody's figured out a way to slide some by."

"Send and receive complete" the tiny box in the corner of the screen read. Karen thought, "Good, only those few pieces of trash to delete and oh, there is one legitimate e-mail. Subject line: Individual Counseling Request. I'll answer this and get to bed." Karen opened the e-mail and read.

It was the lady with the rheumatoid arthritis and ulcerative colitis. A stab of dismay went through Karen's heart as she looked at the date. The woman had responded to her e-mail that she had just sent out—basically today. "This

Lyn has probably been waiting on tenterhooks for my reply for the entire last week. I *have* to keep up with these e-mails somehow."

Karen read the short e-mail requesting further help. She would have her daughter Ruth, who was also her secretary, call her in the morning to set up a time. It was a good thing that Lyn wanted personal help. Ulcerative colitis as well as rheumatoid arthritis could take so many turns that it really was necessary to walk a client through the process on an individual basis.

* * * * * * *

Lyn was at work. The phone interrupted Lyn's concentration as she calculated stock option values.

"Hello, this is Lyn."

"This is Ruth from Karen R. Hurd Nutritional Practice. I understand that you would like to set up an appointment with Karen."

Hooray! The woman had received her e-mail from just last night. "I do. But I won't be able to come to her office. I live in southeastern Wisconsin about thirty minutes south of Milwaukee and she's all the way up by Eau Claire."

"That's not a problem. Karen does many telephone consultations. She'll still be able to help you."

The young woman who had identified herself as Ruth was very reassuring. They arranged a date and time. August fourth, 2004. Maybe then Lyn would begin to get some answers.

CHAPTER 4

The Nuts and Bolts of Ulcerative Colitis

"Hello, Lyn. This is Karen. It's nice to meet you over the phone. I've been looking forward to speaking with you."

The woman's voice was pleasant and confident. Lyn's heart flickered with hope yet again. It had encouraged her so much when she had received that first response to her e-mail. "Your problems are very easy to correct with diet alone." And then when she had set up the consultation time with Ruth, again she had felt that hope. Both of these women seemed so placidly certain that she was fixable. It had been such a relief, especially after receiving the news from the doctor that her condition was a lifelong, incurable disease with periods of exacerbation and remission. Lyn could hear him now. She surely hoped that Karen and Ruth were right and not the doctor.

"I did receive all the paperwork that you sent via e-mail. Thank you for taking the time to fill out those forms for me. They give me more pieces to the puzzle of Lyn Redmond. And the more pieces of the puzzle that I have, the easier it is to solve."

Karen went over the information that Lyn had sent, asking many questions of clarification. By the time Karen finished, Lyn felt that the woman must know not only her entire health picture, but she could probably ascertain her relationship with her husband, boss, and friends! But Lyn was thankful that the woman was digging for all the information that she could unearth. It indicated to Lyn that she would not be receiving a generic quick-fix package to get well, but an individualized plan tailored just to her.

"Lyn, you have written that your top desires for better health are to see ulcerative colitis in remission and to not be so tired all the time."

"Yes," Lyn replied. "I'm desperate. I feel like my life revolves around the restroom; I'm willing to try *anything* you suggest."

Karen laughed. "Well, what I ask you to do won't be too difficult. You won't have to eat fish eyes and lizard tails—it'll just be regular food. It's just the choices in food that you have been making that will need to change. Although during the healing phase, we will emphasize some foods more than others."

Karen continued, "If you don't mind, I'd also like to help you with some of the other problems that you have brought up: the rheumatoid arthritis, the almost-daily headaches, the frequent bladder infections, and finally, I'd like to help you with the infertility."

"You'll be able to help me with all of those, too?" Lyn couldn't keep the incredulity out of her voice.

"Yes, however, the infertility will take the longest and will require your patience for a lengthy period of time—at least a few years, although some of my clients are able to conceive in one year—it depends on the individual situation."

"Do you give out guarantees?" Lyn couldn't help but ask.

Laughing, the woman responded, "No. Only God gives guarantees. I cannot promise you that you will be healed of anything. But I do promise you that I'll do all within my power and knowledge to help you become as healthy as you can be, and *that* usually results in healing from all the problems that you have."

"Okay, I'm ready. Tell me what to do," Lyn said. She had a pen and paper ready and was going to write down everything Karen said.

"I will be very specific in telling you what to do, but first I need to educate you a little in two areas. One is the endocrine system, but the most important one that we need to first address is the gastro-intestinal system. I'd like to stop this craziness of eight to nine bloody stools a day. Also, I want to relieve the cramping that you have with those bowel movements."

Lyn interjected, "Some of them aren't even true bowel movements—they're just blood."

Karen's voice was soft when she responded and held such empathy that Lyn felt like crying. "I know, Lyn. Let's work at stopping this misery." Lyn's mind sobbed—there was a person out there that really cared, that really hurt with her. "I will do whatever this lady says to get better," Lyn thought, "even if she said I did have to eat fish eyes and lizard tails."

Lyn's pen flew as she listened to the detailed explanation. Karen was obviously putting it into layman's terms to help her to understand as much as possible, but it was incredible how much the woman knew about the inner workings of the body.

"There is a large organ called the liver that makes a digestive fluid called bile. Bile is used to break down the fatty foods that you eat. After the bile is made in the liver it is sent to the gall bladder. The gall bladder is located underneath the liver. The liver covers over the gall bladder like a hood. The bile travels down a little pathway called a duct and deposits in the gall bladder. It is stored there until a meal is eaten. When you eat, the gall bladder releases a significant amount of the bile fluid into the duodenum, which is the first part of your small intestine.

"Lyn, I want you to know where your duodenum is. Put your hand on your abdomen, above your belly button and below your sternum. Your sternum is where your rib cage comes together at the front. Is your hand there?"

"Yes, it is," Lyn replied.

"That is your duodenum. Most people identify that place as the stomach, but really it's the small intestine. The stomach is actually underneath your left breast."

Karen continued her explanation. "Once the bile is released into the duodenum it begins to digest the fats that you just consumed. The bile will travel from the duodenum to the jejunum and then the ileum. These are other parts of the small intestine. When the bile reaches the last part of the ileum something very significant happens."

Karen paused. She knew that Lyn was taking notes. She wanted to let her catch up because this point was so important.

"Okay, I'm ready," Lyn said.

"Bile is absorbed in the terminal part of the ileum and returns to the liver from whence it came." Karen waited a moment to make sure Lyn had it written down. "This becomes monumentally important because of another role that the liver plays. Not only does the liver make bile, the liver is the main detoxification organ in the entire body.

"There are other organs that also clean toxins out of the body, but the liver carries the vast majority of the load. The liver deals with some of the most dangerous poisons to which we are exposed. The liver filters fat-soluble trash from the blood."

Karen became animated as she continued. "Once the liver has cleaned these fatty little nasties from the bloodstream, it looks for a place to get rid of them. Really, what should the liver be doing with the trash that it collects? Most people don't think about this, but the liver does. Should the liver put poisons back into the bloodstream? No, that would be ridiculous. It just cleaned them out of the bloodstream. Should the liver somehow transport the trash to the skin and allow it to 'evaporate' out of the body. No, that wouldn't work because the way to transport the trash to the skin would be back through the bloodstream. Well, is there a way to send the trash down to the kidneys and then to the bladder? Is it possible to toss the nasties into the urine? No, that won't work either. There is no connection between the liver and the kidneys or bladder. The kidneys and bladder can only handle water-soluble trash, not fat-soluble trash. No, the liver is going to have to find another exit for its garbage.

"Well, there is that digestive fluid that the liver makes called bile. The bile goes from the liver into the gastro-intestinal tract and will travel the length of that system and YES! It will leave the body in the form of a bowel movement. Perfect! We throw the little nasties into the toilet and flush them away!"

Lyn laughed. "You have an interesting way to explain things."

"I have to. When a person talks about the body it's oftentimes boring, so I try to spice it up a little. If I didn't you would be asleep in a few minutes after I began the explanation."

"I'm glad that you are taking the time to go through this though. It's fascinating," Lyn said.

"I've found that if I don't explain what's going on, the person I'm trying to help will probably not follow through on the things I ask them to do. Knowledge is very powerful, and an understanding of how the body works will help to give them the mental muscle that they need when they are faced with a food that I might put on their 'forbidden list.'"

"Forbidden list?" Lyn questioned with a bit of fearful anticipation edging her voice.

Karen couldn't help laughing. She responded in a mock evil-sounding whisper, "Yes, the forbidden list. You will have one. But that's for later. Don't let your mind go there. You have to learn several more things before we get to the 'lists.'"

"Almost sounds like some type of torture—'the lists,'" Lyn replied.

Karen could hardly talk through her laughter. "Some may see it as torturous, but you'll see that it's not at all bad. And if you heal, what's a little inconvenience for a short time?" Karen stifled her laughter, adopted a serious lecture tone and said, "Back to the books, ma'am. Take good notes.

"You should have noted that the liver puts the fat-soluble toxins it filters from the blood into the digestive fluid bile, sending these foul substances to the gastro-intestinal tract to eventually be deposited in the toilet. But there is this little catch.

"Bile is absorbed in the last part of the small colon! That means that the trash that was tucked away into the bile is *also* absorbed. All of the little nasties go back to the liver with the returning bile! We never got rid of them. Not good.

"The liver says to the returning bile with incredulous anger, 'What in the world are you doing back here!? I sent you down to the gastro-intestinal tract so that you would be thrown into the toilet!'

"The bile stutters its response, 'It's not my fault. Lyn didn't eat anything to make me leave. Uh, you do remember that bile absorbs from the ileum, sir? So, here I am.'

"The liver shouts back, 'Don't lecture me on the absorption of bile. I'm the expert in bile knowledge. Don't you know that I'm the producer of bile! What you don't know is that while you've been monkeying around in the gut for the past several hours, I've been filtering blood and gathering more trash. And *you* have returned with your toxins in tow. Now I am forced to put my recently collected garbage into bile that is already laden with refuse. That will make you especially foul. In fact, twice as foul as you are now.'

"The bile shies away from the liver's rage but is met by the hot words, 'Get over here, you blasted bile. I will have to resend you to the gastro-intestinal tract. Just make sure you get thrown into the toilet this time. You're carrying a double load of trash now. Don't you dare think about coming back!'

"'Uh, yes sir, but…but…it all depends on if Lyn eats…'

"The liver cuts off the protests from the bile and sends it down to the gastro-intestinal tract. But the bile is right, Lyn. If you don't eat the right foods, the bile will be standing on the liver's doorstep again.[1]"

"And will the liver put even more toxins in the bile?" Lyn's question was excellent.

"That's exactly what will happen. The liver will continue to put more and more fat-soluble waste into the bile each time it returns, so it is only a matter of time before the bile is so foul that it has become a literal monster. It comes into contact with your delicate intestinal lining and wreaks havoc. It's like General Sherman marching through the South, burning and destroying as he goes. Your bile has become so foul that it creates irritation and eventually sores in the gastro-intestinal tract. The sores can become so bad that they

---

[1] See appendix for further remarks and references.

open up and bleed. If the sores and bleeding occur in the small intestine, we call it Crohn's disease. If the sores and bleeding occur in the large intestine, we call it ulcerative colitis."

"That's what I have then—bile irritation that has gone so far as to create sores in my large intestine," Lyn said.

"That's it," Karen answered.

"But the doctors told me it was an auto-immune problem that diet could not help," Lyn protested.

Karen responded in a gentle voice, "They are well-meaning, Lyn. They are trying their best, but they will confess to you that the auto-immune answer is only a theory. Mine also is only a theory. Everyone has to work from some sort of hypothesis. Then as we apply the indicated answers based on our hypotheses, theories are proven and research eventually backs it up. I have yet much to explain to you on the auto-immune theory as that is a major bug-a-boo in your understanding of rheumatoid arthritis. That subject I must address today also, as I want to help you with rheumatoid arthritis as well as your ulcerative colitis. But first we have to finish the bile story."

"I am extremely curious what food I have to eat to make my bile go into the toilet," Lyn responded.

"Ah, it's a good thing that you're curious. That'll make it easier for you when I require you to eat this food six times a day until you are well. But I'm going to keep you in suspense a little longer until you understand just a bit more.

"In the digestion process, bile will bind to foods. Bile has a certain affinity, or a liking, for some foods. Normally bile is not too choosy about what it combines with, taking or leaving whatever happens to land in the duodenum. But there is one particular substance that bile falls head-over-heels in love with. So much so that it will unbind with whatever substance it is currently bound to and rush to bind with this particular food. That food is soluble fiber."

"What kind of food is soluble fiber?" Lyn was definitely curious.

"Can't spill the beans all at once, can I?" Karen said with barely suppressed laughter. "I'll tell you in just a minute."

"Okay, I'll be patient," Lyn answered.

"Soluble fiber is just as strongly attracted to bile. Imagine this, Lyn." Karen continued in a love-song type of voice. "The soluble fiber enters the duodenum from the stomach. The bile enters from the gall bladder. They see each other from across a crowded duodenum and rush into each other's arms, forsaking any others that they might have bonded with. They make nuptial vows promising to remain together for the rest of their lives."

"Is that really what happens?" Lyn asked.

"Actually, yes. But if I explained it in terms of ionic bonds and covalent bonds, I'd have to give you a short course in chemistry, and I didn't know if you wanted to do that today. So it's best to say that the bile and soluble fiber get married and there is no such word as divorce."

Lyn was very interested. "I'm all ears. Keep going."

"The happily married bile and soluble fiber travel gaily through the intestinal tract. They pass through the jejunum and finally arrive at the ileum. At that point the bile turns to the soluble fiber and says, 'My partner and dearest friend, it has been wonderful journeying through the gastro-intestinal tract with you. Now I will take you on a honeymoon excursion. For the last several years I have returned to the liver at this point. So we'll go there together.'

"The soluble fiber responds with hesitancy in her voice, 'Um, there was something that I forgot to tell you about myself before we got married up there in the duodenum. Uh ...I can't cross the intestinal barrier, not here, not anywhere.' Then the soluble fiber's voice takes on a firmer tone with her husband. 'Remember, we're married and there is no such word as divorce? Well, I'm going into the toilet and you're coming with me!' And off they go into the sewer system in the form of a bowel movement.

"I can't resist telling you what one of my clients said to me at this point during my bile and soluble fiber illustration. He said, 'I guess that's what is meant when you hear that someone's marriage has gone down the drain.'"

Lyn laughed. "Okay, okay. But I'm on pins and needles. Obviously I'm going to have to eat this soluble fiber. What food is it that has this wonderful ingredient?"

"I gave you a hint before." Karen didn't try to suppress the chuckle now.

"I must have missed it," Lyn replied. "I truly don't know."

"Beans," Karen answered.

"Beans? What kind of beans?" was Lyn's surprised reply.

"Beans—like pinto, kidney, garbanzo, Great Northern, navy, lentils, limas." Karen's voice took up a chant-like rhythm as she continued, "black beans, brown beans, white beans, red beans," now her voice switched to a different meter, "black-eyed peas, yellow-eyed peas, pigeon peas, green split peas, yellow split peas." Karen hesitated, "I think you probably have the idea of the type of beans now. Please note though that green beans and wax beans are not to be considered legumes. They are vegetables. Also soy beans and peanuts are not to be regarded as legumes. They're goobers. They don't have the soluble fiber in a high enough concentration for them to be considered for our purposes."

"Goobers?" Lyn couldn't help asking.

"Cool term, isn't it? I've always liked it too. But I can't spend any time on goobers today because we'll be on the phone for hours. And I still have to tell you about rheumatoid arthritis and . . ." Karen's voice went teasingly sinister, "...the lists."

Lyn laughed. "Okay, I'll curb my curiosity about goobers and pay attention."

"Thank you, ma'am. Onward we go. The beans that are loaded with soluble fiber will marry the bile and force the exit of this foul substance which has been burning holes in your gut. The liver will rejoice and make brand-new bile as none is returned from the ileum. By the way, I'd like to spin out another thread which we won't cover but you should have this floating around in the back of your mind—the liver makes bile out of triglycerides and low density lipoproteins—what we term 'bad cholesterol'. When the liver makes new bile it pulls this heart-clogging fat from the bloodstream and turns it into bile which you'll marry to soluble fiber and toss into the toilet."

"You mean that a person can lower cholesterol by eating beans?" Lyn was catching on.

"Exactly," Karen replied. "And here's another piece of information that you need to know. Bile that has circulated over and over again becomes thicker and even tar-like after a time. It will form residues, sludge, and even gall stones causing gall bladder disease. As the liver makes new bile, this residual old bile will be dissolved and removed, but it will take around six to ten weeks for this to occur—and that's at fifty-plus grams of soluble fiber per day. Sometimes it takes longer—but not for many."

"Whoa, slow down. People with gall bladder problems can be helped by this also?"

"Absolutely. But this is another thread in the tapestry of health that I won't explain today. The reason I'm giving you this piece of information is for you to understand that you also will have some bile residue which is injurious to the intestinal tract; therefore, your ulcerative colitis will not be cured in one week. It will take us several weeks. But each day that passes you'll be better and eventually you can be completely well.

"We also have to allow time for the existing ulcers to heal. They are sores like any other. They will close up and disappear altogether in time. Actually, it won't take too much time for that part. Ulcers in the gastro-intestinal tract mend rapidly. We just have to give them a chance to heal by not washing nasty bile over them and not scratching them with foods that act like scouring brushes. So I'll be very strict with your diet in the beginning to facilitate the healing of your ulcers, but we'll go ahead and start tossing out bile right away using the beans. Soluble fiber won't irritate the sores. It actually soothes them."

Lyn interrupted, "I'm ready for 'the lists.'"

"No. Not yet. I know this seems like a ton of information, but I still have to tell you about how we are going to beat rheumatoid arthritis."

"Wait a minute. I want to start on a clean sheet." Karen could hear Lyn tearing pages off a tablet. "Okay, go."

CHAPTER 5

Some New Thoughts about Rheumatoid Arthritis

"Rheumatoid arthritis is one of the most misunderstood health problems that there is. The biggest stumbling block is that the majority of people are operating under a wrong hypothesis. Wait a minute, let me make this clear: *I* believe they are operating under the wrong assumption," Karen said.

Lyn interrupted. "My doctors told me that rheumatoid arthritis was caused by a dysfunction of my immune system. They called it an autoimmune disease."

"This is exactly my point. They, unfortunately, are operating under a theory that has not been proven true. In fact, all evidence points to the fact that the theory of rheumatoid arthritis being an autoimmune disease is more than *not* true. Not only is it mistaken, but when we apply solutions using an incorrect theory as a basis, we can actually cause more harm than good. It is sad for me to report that this is exactly what I believe has happened with rheumatoid arthritis."

Karen gave Lyn a minute to absorb her last statements and then said quietly, "Doctors are not trying to mislead people. They are truly doing their very best to try to help people. But sometimes we, as humans, get going down a wrong path and it's hard to see that maybe the path we're on isn't the right one. It's even harder to see when the majority of our friends and colleagues are on the same path as we are.

"In that same vein, I'm fully aware that I myself may be traveling a path that is wrong. So I am constantly re-evaluating my position. Are the things

I'm doing helpful? If my theory is true, I should be seeing results. If I'm not seeing the proper results then my theory may be faulty and need to be reworked. And most importantly, am I causing any harm?

"'Above all else, do no harm.'" Karen whispered to herself those words of the famed Hippocratic oath that all physicians were taught to uphold. One of the deepest desires in her heart was to free people from the physical ailments that crippled them. She knew that mirrored the desire of the hearts of doctors also. "At least my tools of healing cause no harm. I am thankful of that."

"Karen, I missed the last thing you said. I think our connection is going bad."

"Sorry, Lyn, that was my fault. I wasn't speaking very loudly. Lyn, I want to tell you a little story. It's something that I learned when I was a young officer in the U.S. Army at the Military Intelligence School in Ft. Huachuca, Arizona.

"It was the summer of 1980 and I sat in a large classroom with many other second lieutenants for our Officer Basic Training Course. It was hot and the swamp coolers were not keeping up. The walls were painted a light green color which helped a little in the suggestion of coolness, but as I glanced at the young lieutenant next to me wiping sweat off his brow, I remember thinking that at least the classroom training was not as broiling as the field training. We were scheduled for another bout of that starting the next day. The topic for the class this particular afternoon was Final Protective Fires and was being taught by a major that I had not seen before. I was prepared to listen to this teaching of military tactics again. I had already had this class in my ROTC education in college, but a refresher was always good.

"'Class,' the quick sharp voice of the major tatted like the Morse code that we had recently learned, 'if you hear nothing else I say today, hear this.'

"I sat up a little straighter. No officer had begun a class like this before. I was interested in what the man was going to say.

"'More soldiers have been killed and we have lost more battles because of this one simple mistake.' The major paused to make sure he had the entire class's attention before continuing. 'The officer-in-charge failed to change his battle plan.'

"The major didn't need to worry that he didn't have the class's attention. We were all ears. He then gave us the explanation that we were waiting for.

"'If your back is against a wall and you are forced to call for final protective fires, NEVER dismiss the possibility that there may be other options.'

"I need to let you know, Lyn, that when a company commander—or any officer-in-charge is forced to call in final protective fires, it means that the unit is facing overwhelming forces and is about to be wiped off the face of the earth. The point of final protective fires is to provide a last wall of protection that allows the maneuver commander to have a short space of time to readjust his plan—if it's not too late—before the entire unit goes down to the grave. It's a desperation measure.

"The major continued, 'Our most brilliant military geniuses have always been noted for their ability to come up with options that are outside the norm. On the other hand, the average officer, once he sees that his battle plan is not working, calls for final protective fires while giving the troops the rah-rah speech of "Come on, men, we can do it. A little longer, a little harder and we'll beat the enemy back" when all the while he knows that they are about to go to their deaths despite their efforts. Never resign yourself to what *you* see as the inevitable. There is always more to see than what you think there is. Instead of fighting harder, fight smarter. Figure out a new plan that could possibly work to get your troops out of there.'

"The major paused for a long moment as he looked at us with cold eyes that snapped and then said in a steely voice, 'When your battle plan is failing, lieutenant, change your battle plan and final protective fires may never become necessary.'

"I sat there in one of those rare moments of realization—the type of moment when a light bulb blazes in a person's head and they know that they've heard something that they will never forget. The major went on instructing us in how to call in the artillery fire, but I was not focused on that. The man was right about changing battle plans! But it wasn't just a principle that should be applied to warfare; it was a principle that should be applied to everyday life. How many times had I, or people that I knew, had a plan to accomplish some task and no matter how hard I tried or they tried the goal was never reached?

"Lyn, do you see my point? When our battle plan is failing, we shouldn't say, 'I'll try again, but I'll try harder this time.' Or 'I'll do the battle plan longer.' Good grief! The battle plan has failed. The methodology that we were using doesn't work. Instead of doing the same stupid plan over again—which will result in the same dismal failure—throw the battle plan out the window. Go back to the drawing board and formulate a new battle plan. And if that one fails, formulate yet another battle plan until one is found that will allow us to win the war. People keep using the same battle plan over and over again hoping that 'this time' it might work."

Karen paused and then said, "Change your battle plan, lieutenant."

Lyn's voice was quiet as she replied, "I do see. I have been doing a battle plan for my rheumatoid arthritis that hasn't worked, but instead of changing my plan, I've continued to do the same strategy, hoping that it might work somehow. And it hasn't. It has *never* worked. I still have rheumatoid arthritis." Lyn's voice grew indignant. "But I knew that rheumatoid arthritis was incurable so I figured that what I was doing was the only plan there was!"

Karen responded in a calm voice, "That's how everyone feels when they are convinced that there are no solutions—that their fate is inevitable. Remember there is always more to see than what we think there is. Lyn, you have set up final protective fires, trying to stave off the onslaught that has threatened to overwhelm you. But what you really need to do is to change your battle plan."

"I guess that's why I'm talking to you today. I need a new strategy," Lyn replied.

Karen said, "I will be the first one to return to the drawing board and suggest a new battle plan if the plan I give you does not work. It has worked for many others, but if for some reason it fails you, I will apply myself diligently in finding a health strategy that will work for you."

"Thank you," Lyn answered.

"Now, you must understand several things before I can tell you the plan to resolve the trouble that you are in. First and foremost, I do not believe that rheumatoid arthritis is an autoimmune disease. I cannot swallow the theory that the immune system is so skewed that it has turned traitor and is attacking the very cells that it is supposed to be protecting. Instead, I believe we have a normal response from the immune system, but we have not identified the real culprit.

"There is this simple law of nature. You will be very familiar with it. When two surfaces are rubbed together the force of friction is created. Lyn, please rub your hands together. If you have to put the phone down to do it, I'll wait."

After a moment Karen asked, "What happened when you rubbed your hands together?"

Lyn's reply was quick, "They got warmer."

"That is the result of the force of friction. Friction always results in heat. Imagine if you continued to rub your hands together for two hours. How would they feel?"

"My hands would be sore and irritated."

"Imagine rubbing them together non-stop for days on end. How would they feel?"

"Incredibly painful."

"Exactly. In fact, after several days the damage to your hands would be so severe that you might not even be alive anymore. The skin will have rubbed off and you very well may have bled to death. That is the destructive power of friction. Friction creates heat and heat applied over time, even in small amounts, will damage human tissue."

"That makes sense," Lyn said.

"If this law of nature is true, why isn't every single human dead?"

Karen did not wait for a response from Lyn. "Without some intervening factor, we all would be dead before we even left the womb. We are one mass of movement. Our joints are rubbing together almost constantly. Think about it. Your shoulders are moving, your knees, your ankles, your elbows, the joints in your hands and feet, your vertebrae, the huge mandible which is your jaw bone is creaking up and down on its hinges. Even if you were perfectly still and didn't move a joint in your entire body, you would still have the blood rubbing against your arteries, veins, and capillaries as it passes through. Your heart is beating against your chest; your lungs are inflating against the thoracic wall; you will never stop moving until you draw your final breath.

"Movement always means that there will be friction. Friction means heat. Heat means damage to human tissue." Karen paused to emphasize the next statement. "But there is a mitigating factor. That factor is corticosteroids.

"Corticosteroids are very powerful hormones that reduce and reverse the negative effects of friction.[2] They prevent the tissues from becoming inflamed and sore as a result of the rubbing force of friction. Corticosteroids are like the grease between the parts on a mechanical contraption. We all know that if metal parts rub against one another that the friction causes the metal to heat and expand. Then the parts lock up and are not able to move anymore. That is exactly what arthritis is. The more we rub, the more heat we have, the more swelling we'll have and then our parts eventually lock up and we can't move. We call it all kinds of names like bursitis, tendonitis, fibromyalgia, polymyalgia rheumatica, but most commonly we call it arthritis. All the other terms just describe where the inflammation is—in the bursa, in the muscle, in the tendon, etcetera. All of these problems and even more—but I won't bore you today with those—are all caused by the very same thing: rubbing without sufficient grease between the moving parts."

Lyn interjected, "You've described exactly how I feel, like a piece of creaking machinery that is about to lock up. Is this related to cortisone shots? My doctor has talked about those."

"Absolutely related. A cortisone shot is just putting a corticosteroid at the place of inflammation. It's a local measure to reduce the pain of arthritis.

"So you can see the solution is to get the grease back between the parts—which we can and will do without having to take cortisone shots or corticosteroids in pill form. But before I tell you why your body hasn't been

---

2 See appendix for further remarks and references.

producing enough corticosteroid and how in the world we're going to get it to make enough, I want to finish addressing this autoimmune business.

"If there is insufficient grease, and I'm going to call it corticosteroid from here on out because that is what the grease is, the rubbing continues to aggravate the tissue until there is inflammation and literal damage to the human cells. Of course, this makes for pain. We are literally rubbing ourselves raw!

"Now, here is the next piece. When you have a sore, a scrape, or a scratch, what system do you think will be called in to fix it?"

Karen waited for Lyn's response. After a brief moment Lyn ventured, "The immune system?"

"You got it. The immune system is responsible for mending the damage that occurs in the human body. So the immune system rushes to the scene of the crime to begin to repair the hurting flesh. But you must understand how the immune system works. It starts the healing process by encircling the damaged area with a bubble of fluid. This fluid will isolate the injury while the flesh is being mended.

"But, Lyn, if we put fluid in an area where it is not normally supposed to be, that will make *more* pain. We will put *more* pressure on the nerve endings that communicate pain to our brains."

"Nerve endings?" Lyn interrupted. "Where do they fit in?"

"Nerves communicate messages to the brain. If nerves or nerve endings are pressed in any way, they will send a message to the brain that says PAIN.

"Here's the double whammy. Not only do we have the original pain occurring from the rubbing of surfaces without enough corticosteroid, but the immune system is adding to the misery by pumping in fluid in spaces that are too little to contain it without terrible discomfort."

"I thought the immune system was supposed to help the body," Lyn commented.

"It is. And this addition of a protective bubble of fluid acts like the truest friend that there could ever be."

"I don't get it. How can adding to pain be a beneficial thing?"

"Lyn, let's pretend that you are chopping vegetables for dinner tonight. As you are working on the celery, the paring knife slips and you accidentally cut your left index finger. The cut is not especially deep but it's on the tip, right in the center of the inside pad. It bleeds a little. You run water over the top of it, and you pat it off with a paper towel to dry it. Then you put an adhesive bandage on the cut."

"Okay," Lyn said a bit cautiously.

"You finish chopping the vegetables and complete the rest of the dinner preparation. But where is your injured finger during this process? Are you using it as normal?"

"No, I would be holding it up and out of the way while I worked," Lyn replied.

"Yes. You work with nine fingers instead of ten because if you used that injured finger there would be pain involved as you apply pressure to the cut *and because it is surrounded by a small influx of fluid that the immune system furnishes, you will be especially sensitive to pressure and therefore pain.*

"Let me take this illustration just a bit further so that you will understand the next part which becomes very important when we formulate a solution for healing based on this theory. It is especially vital to know as that solution will demand that we depart from the traditional medical doctor's recommendations.

"As your cut heals through the next day or so, you find that it's not wise for you to use that finger. You tried removing the bandage but replaced it with another because every time you caught your finger on something—which was often because of the location of the cut—the thin little scab that had formed on the area was pulled off, making the injured area bleed again. Also, it was painful each time you touched anything with that finger. Pressure applied to an area that has extra fluid that normally doesn't belong there always creates pain. The pain constantly reminds you to leave that finger alone and not use it until it heals.

"If you would continue to use your injured finger, the cut would be reopened again and again as you tore off the scab. That would delay the healing of your finger indefinitely. In time, the immune system might be able to get enough repair work done, despite the overwhelming odds against it that the wound would finally close and 'heal.' But understand the immune system was so hindered in the process that it would be unable to do its normally superb job. The mending is done, but done roughly. Now on your finger you carry a scar. The original damage was not really that bad; a scar should never have developed unless the cut had been extremely deep or wide. Your cut was neither, but you develop scar tissue because you kept re-injuring the area.

"It's like the child who has a mosquito bite. He scratches the bite and breaks it open. Then like children often do, he picks the scab off. Another scab forms, and the child picks that scab off. His mother keeps telling him to quit picking at the scab because it'll form a scar which indeed it will. If the child leaves it alone, there will be no scar."

Lyn couldn't help but ask, "Karen, are you saying that I could be forming scar tissue inside my body, on a joint?"

Karen's voice was full of compassion as she replied, "Yes. The official word for scar tissue found on arthritic joints is *pannus*. Scar tissue is never elastic like normal tissue. It is tough and stiff. Therefore it limits the motion of the joint. It can even cause the drawing up of a joint which can cause deformity. You may have seen older people with arthritis that have gnarled hands. Those knobby hands are caused by scar tissue on the joint."

Lyn's voice was faint, "Oh."

Karen finished the explanation. "The immune system is our friend because it puts fluid around the injured area to create more pain so that we won't be tempted to use the area. An undisturbed area is far easier to heal and will not be so likely to demand the use of fibrous scar tissue to seal it.

"So the occurrence of arthritis in my theory is this:

1. The joints rub together without enough corticosteroid to negate frictional damage—we feel stiff and sore.

2. The immune system arrives to repair the frictional damage.

3. The immune system places a protective layer of fluid around the injured area—we feel even more pain.

4. We continue to use the injured area, ignoring the pain or using pain-killing medications to mask over the difficulty, and the immune system has to work harder to heal the continually re-injured area.

5. Not being able to work unhindered, the immune system is forced to rougher healing methods. Scar tissue begins to form."

Karen could hear Lyn's pen scratching across her paper as she rapidly took notes. Karen waited another moment and then said, "Lyn, have you ever read murder mysteries?"

"Sure."

"How often have you read this type of scenario? 'The assassin finishes his foul work and drops the blood-stained knife on the floor when he hears a man calling from the foot of the stairs. "Honey, are you up there?" The criminal quickly opens the window and climbs onto the roof, closing the window behind him just before the husband enters the room and discovers the atrocity. The murderer jumps from the roof making his escape unnoticed by the distraught husband. The husband picks up the murder weapon, staring in horror at the tool that has robbed him of the most precious thing he had in life. He stumbles to the phone on the bedside table and calls the police. After a few moments he is relieved to hear the running footfalls on the stairs. The police burst through the door and find him still holding the murder weapon.'

"Lyn, who did the murder?"

"The man who escaped."

"And the police? Who will they think did the murder?"

"The husband."

"Yes. The police will begin their investigation but find no fingerprints on the knife but the husband's. Unbeknownst to anyone, the murderer had taken precautions and worn gloves. The husband violently proclaims his innocence but the pieces of the puzzle don't fit together in his favor. The husband is indicted and convicted. It's all too obvious. The husband killed her."

"But there is always other evidence before a conviction is made," Lyn protested.

"You're right, there is. And in this case after much investigation, it was found that the husband had recently taken out a large life insurance policy on his wife. His insipid claims that he had taken out the policy because of his brother's advice (who had just lost his wife to cancer) held no weight with the judge. Also the fact that he had a public argument with his wife the night before at a party was used as evidence against him. The judge considered it an open and shut case. Punishment was meted out to the killer, who obviously was the husband.

"Now, Lyn, bear with me as I draw the net for you. The immune system is blamed for arthritis because it is caught holding the murder weapon. The immune system did not create the damage that it arrived on the scene to heal. But it's hard to believe that the immune system is innocent when there are signs to indicate its guilt. We have antinuclear antibodies and the Rheumatoid Factor as well as sedimentation rates that indicate the immune system is at work in this crime. Unfortunately, the authorities didn't know that those blood and urine tests only indicate the presence of an actively working immune system—they don't necessarily indicate culpability."

"So the immune system is blamed for the crime," Lyn stated more than questioned.

"Yes. And if the immune system is at fault then the obvious cure is to squelch the immune system. Knock it down. Lock it up. Disable it." Karen waited a minute before concluding. "Lyn, that's exactly the current medical method used to 'control' arthritis. The doctors freely admit that there is no cure because they can see that the immuno-suppressant drugs don't take away arthritis. They just help control the pain. The scarring and deformity will still occur."

"I see." Lyn's voice was flat. "If the immune system is not allowed to function properly, it won't put the protective fluid around the injured area, so a person won't feel the pain like they would have with a fully functioning immune system."

"Yes."

Karen waited. This was so difficult for people. So hard to accept that the path one was traveling may not have been the right one. In fact, that very path might have caused more harm than good.

"Karen?" Lyn's voice sounded thin over the phone lines.

"Yes?"

"If your theory is correct, then the medications that I have been using have only served to aggravate my overall situation. Is that right?"

"Some of your medications are steroids. They mimic the activity of the corticosteroids that you are naturally supposed to make to reduce the everyday inflammation of the joints. They do perpetuate your arthritis, but in a different way that I have yet to explain. At least you were not prescribed Remicade or methotrextrate. Those medications are specifically targeted to disable your immune system. The steroidal drugs directly reduce inflammation and only indirectly disable your immune system."

"You mean the Vioxx?" Lyn asked.

"No, I actually mean one of the medications you were prescribed for the ulcerative colitis. Remember how you said that when you began treating the ulcerative colitis that somehow your rheumatoid arthritis improved?"

"Yes. The rheumatoid arthritis got better, more than it ever had with the Vioxx," Lyn replied.

"That's because one the medications for the ulcerative colitis is a steroid. The Vioxx is not."

"Then is Vioxx the type of drug that disables my immune system?"

"No, not directly. Not like the immuno-suppressant medications. Vioxx is a non-steroidal anti-inflammatory drug. These types of medications are commonly called NSAIDs."

"You said 'not directly'. What does that mean?"

"Vioxx is not a body-friendly substance. Even though it is not targeted to squelch the immune system, it does knock it back by stimulating the production of the hormone adrenalin.[3]"

"How does it do that?" Lyn asked.

"When a drug or foreign substance enters the bloodstream, it will be filtered out in the normal manner. However, oftentimes the brain directs the endocrine system to speed the filtration process because the foreign substance is particularly dangerous. The more aggravating the drug, the bigger demand the brain will place on the endocrine system to speed filtration."

"So the endocrine system filters out the bad stuff in our blood?" Lyn asked.

"No, it doesn't. The liver and the kidneys do that work. But the liver, which does the vast majority of the work that is affecting Lyn Redmond's health at this time, will only filter two to four quarts of blood per minute."

"Wow. That's amazing," Lyn said.

"It is. But as amazing as this filtering feat is, the brain is not satisfied. Nasties need to be cleaned out faster! So the message reaches the endocrine system that we need to increase the speed of the blood flowing through the liver.

"The liver is a static organ—in other words it does not actively reach out, grabbing bad guys out of the bloodstream—it simply filters out the offending substances as the blood passes through it. If we have to filter faster, we must make the blood flow faster through the liver."

---

[3] See appendix for further remarks and references.

"How is that done?" Lyn asked.

"By the production of the hormone adrenalin. Adrenalin is one of the most powerful vasoconstrictive substances that there is. An adrenalin release makes our blood vessels shrink up. That means there is less space for the blood to travel through. If there is less space and the same amount of blood, then the blood is forced to travel faster. That means more blood pushed through the liver more quickly. This is exactly what the brain has demanded. Faster filtration.

"It's very similar to a garden hose. Imagine trying to water a bed of flowers with a hose that is ten feet away from you. The water flows out of the end of the hose right at your feet. However, if you put your thumb across the nozzle of the hose, closing off some of the opening, the same amount of water is forced to exit through a smaller space. The pressure of the water is increased to the point that it can shoot across that ten feet span with no problem. That's the same principle that the body uses. Constrict the blood vessels and the blood is forced to travel faster."

"But how does faster filtration disable my immune system? Wouldn't taking the junk out of the bloodstream help the immune system?" Lyn asked.

"It's not the filtration process that slows the immune system. And certainly overall, taking the garbage out of the bloodstream is helpful to the immune system. But it's the production of adrenalin that causes the problems," Karen replied. "Adrenalin always lowers immune system function."

"That's not good. I'm an adrenalin junkie," said Lyn.

"Tell me something else shrouded in mystery," Karen said laughing. "Lyn Redmond, the history you gave me of the woman of drive and determination that you are screams of high adrenalin production! You are very funny." Karen was laughing so hard that she wasn't able to talk for a moment.

Lyn was laughing too. "You make me feel better already. I must not be that difficult to fix if you can laugh about it."

"Okay. I'm recovered," Karen said, still fighting down the chuckles, "And yes, you are easy to fix."

"That's so hard for me to believe," Lyn said. "I've been told for so long that it's impossible to cure my conditions."

"It's not impossible. But you don't have to believe blindly. Whether you believe it or not, the proof is in the pudding." Karen began laughing again.

"Now, why are you laughing?" demanded Lyn with false indignation as she herself was having a hard time not joining in. Karen's laughter was infectious.

"I'm not laughing at you, but me. 'Pudding' is not something that I recommend that anyone eat. That expression is one I'll have to learn to strike from my repertoire of clichés. I also frequently use 'Put that in your pipe and smoke it,' and I'll have to learn to eliminate that one too."

Lyn was laughing now. She needed to laugh more often. It felt really good to truly enjoy something. Hope flared in her heart as she thought that it might be possible to feel well enough that she could laugh easily again. This woman seemed to know what she was talking about. Maybe, just maybe, she could be well again.

"Okay, okay," Karen stifled her mirth. "I'll get back to business. I must seriously finish explaining to you how the NSAIDs contribute to lowered immunity." She cleared her throat and began again.

"Remember that the presence of threatening substances in the bloodstream cause an adrenalin release. The adrenalin makes the filtration of the offending party occur more rapidly. The brain is satisfied that all that can be done is being done. But adrenalin squelches the immune system. In fact, adrenalin steps very heavily on the immune system."

"Wow. I've never known that," Lyn said.

"Don't feel badly. Most people don't know that. When I get to the 'lists' I'll tell you other substances that cause this same response. Unfortunately they are prolific in the American diet."

"But why would adrenalin squelch the immune system? It's a natural substance that our own body is making," Lyn asked.

"Lyn, let's pretend that we live in medieval times. You are my avowed enemy, and I am yours. We both happen to be sword masters. We meet in conflict and both draw our swords, finally putting our hatred towards one another to the blade. I am determined to kill you, and you are determined to make this day the last one that I will draw breath.

"We fight in well-executed moves that become more rapid and arduous. After some time you spin on your heel making a plunge for my right side but at the last moment you abort and slash left. I'm not prepared for that move and block to the right leaving my left side exposed. I twist as I see your tactic a moment too late. You miss my torso but leave a large gash in my upper left arm.

"I will not feel any pain. I cannot *afford* to feel pain at this point. If my arm hurt because of that searing and burning slash, I would, without thinking, grab my arm and cry out. But if I did that you would quickly deal me the death blow. Instead, I continue to fight without missing a step. It's as if you had not even injured me.

"This is called the fight and flight response. It's the natural defense mechanism of the body to promote survival. Can you guess the name of the substance that is our fight and flight hormone?"

"It's not a guess. I know the answer. Adrenalin," Lyn answered.

"And adrenalin has to suppress the immune system so that we might live," Karen said. "If the immune system is allowed to work as it is programmed to work, we would immediately have protective layers of fluid placed around the injured arm so the healing process could begin. This additional fluid would put pressure on the nerve endings—communicating pain. We cannot afford to feel pain at that time. We must apply all of our attention to saving our skin. Therefore, the immune system's services are not wanted."

"Is that why I've heard that people who survive a car wreck don't feel pain until later?"

"Yes. And anyone that has ever been in a physical fight will tell you that they felt no pain with their injuries—until later—after the fight was over."

Lyn needed to know something else that had been puzzling her for some time. "Karen, is that why I don't feel the arthritis when I'm angry or super-involved in some project?"

"Yes, ma'am. Any adrenalin release also causes a simultaneous corticosteroid release. The corticosteroid takes away the pain. When a person is angry, they release adrenalin and the accompanying corticosteroids. When a person is producing a large amount of adrenalin to work on an important project, the corticosteroid levels are also increased which results in a reduction of inflammation."

Lyn put it together as she wrote it down in her notes, "So releases of adrenalin for any cause take pain away. And the drug Vioxx, even though it is meant to reduce inflammation only, also works at suppressing my immune system because it causes an adrenalin response."

"Yes, but that medication or any NSAID's effect on the immune system does not hold a candle to the big boys like Remicade or methotrexate. There are also Imuran and a few others that I had not mentioned to you earlier that are also immuno-suppressant drugs."

Karen paused. "And Lyn, there's something else I have to tell you about the Vioxx." She took a breath and said, "It can cause stomach and intestinal problems."

Lyn's voice was incredulous, "You're kidding."

"I am not. Here, I'll read it to you directly from the PDR. It's a huge book that documents every medication on the market, what it does, and what the side effects are."

"What does PDR stand for?"

"Oh, that means Physicians Desk Reference." There was a pause while Karen turned to find the appropriate page in the book. "Here it is, Vioxx. I quote.

"'Warning: Serious gastrointestinal toxicity such as bleeding, ulceration, and perforation of the stomach, small intestine or large intestine, can occur at any time, with or without warning symptoms, in patients treated with non-steroidal anti-inflammatory drugs (NSAIDs).'"[4]

There was silence on the other end of the phone line. Then in a small voice Lyn asked, "What does that book say about Celebrex?"

"Celebrex carries exactly the same warning."

"But Karen, you told me that my ulcerative colitis was caused by nasty bile eating away at my intestinal tract. Now, I find out that the medications I was taking for my rheumatoid arthritis probably caused it."

Karen replied quietly, "Your ulcerative colitis was caused by nasty bile, Lyn. It's the liver that is primarily responsible for clearing both the Celebrex and Vioxx. The liver places the mostly metabolized Celebrex and Vioxx that it collects from the bloodstream into your bile for disposal. Your bile is deposited into your gastro-intestinal tract. Without soluble fiber the bile absorbs at the terminal ileum and returns to the liver with the metabolized Celebrex and Vioxx in tow. The liver will dump yet more of the NSAIDs into the bile. It's not long before the bile is so noxious that it tears up the intestinal tract."

"Oh," Lyn said. "I thought that the medications would directly irritate my colon when I swallowed the pills."

"It's possible, but not the likely conclusion. I'll be able to prove that to you when we get to the lists."

"How will you be able to do that?"

"You'll still need to take the Vioxx, for a time, to control your arthritic pain. Your healing from the rheumatoid arthritis will take longer than the healing from the ulcerative colitis. By eating the soluble fiber in the amounts necessary to remove bile we will cure your ulcerative colitis *while you are yet taking the Vioxx.*"

---

[4] Physicians Desk Reference (2005). New Jersey: Thompson, pg. 2174.

"I see," Lyn replied. "If my ulcerative colitis heals by throwing out the bile while I am still taking the NSAID, then we will know that it was the bile causing my gastro-intestinal problem—not swallowing a pill that landed on my stomach and burned a hole in it while the pill dissolved."

"You got it," Karen replied.

6

CHAPTER 6

Not Enough Grease

"Lyn, you are not producing enough corticosteroid. So we have to ask, 'why not?' Why can't Lyn Redmond make enough grease to keep her parts moving easily?"

"Yeah, I want to know that too," said Lyn.

Karen said, "Corticosteroids are made in the adrenal glands—the same glands that produce all your adrenalin."

"You're kidding."

"Nope. I'm not kidding. Corticosteroids are made in the outlying tissue of the adrenal glands. These little adrenal guys sit on top of your kidneys like small caps. The adrenals produce many hormones for us. But right now we'll look at the hormones produced in the cortex of the adrenals. The cortex is the outlying tissue of the gland. We call the hormones that this part of the gland makes 'corticosteroids' because they are made in the cortex.

"There are several functions of corticosteroids. But one of the major jobs of corticosteroids is to reduce inflammation. Here is the important thing to note: if the adrenal glands become fatigued they will not produce adequate amounts of the hormones that they are assigned to make. Think about it. If you become tired because you have been putting in too many hours at work, or because you have not been getting all your sleep, are you able to function as well?"

Lyn's answer was a simple, "No."

"But you will still go to work and accomplish something even if you are dragging and not as perky as you normally would be with adequate rest?" Karen persisted.

"Yes, I would go to work anyway. But the quality of work and the amount of work that I could achieve would be noticeably less," replied Lyn.

"And so it is with the adrenal glands. If they have been 'put under the gun' so to speak, they will not perform at optimum."

"But isn't this detectable on some sort of blood test? Can't a physician tell if the adrenals are under-functioning?" Lyn asked.

"It's not that easy. The amount of adrenal hormones produced fluctuates so widely in the space of even a few seconds that establishing a 'normal' range has been strictly an exercise in inaccuracy. And even if we didn't have these second-by-second changes in adrenal hormone production, we have this additional catch: every person produces hormones at a level that is specifically necessary for them. Some people are genetically wired to produce higher amounts of the adrenal hormones than others. So what may be normal for you would be a high amount for someone else and vice versa. We can measure the amount of adrenal hormones in the blood at a given moment in time, but the interpretation of the data is unreliable."

"So even if I tested in the 'normal' range it may be abnormal for me?"

"Exactly. And keep in mind that your adrenal demands change by the second. If you are upset about something, you'll need more adrenal hormones. If you are doing more physical movement at that particular moment in time, you'll need more adrenal hormones. If you are working on an urgent project, you'll need more adrenal hormones. Many things affect the demand of adrenal hormones including what you just ate, what you have just inhaled, your menstrual cycle, and even what you have just thought!"

"Oh, my!" Lyn responded.

"It is complicated. That's one of the reasons why this theory of mine is so overlooked. We as a medical society like hard and fast answers; we do not easily allow for nebulous bodily functions that can't be measured accurately. Maybe someday we'll have a diagnostic test to prove this, but right now it doesn't exist."

"Okay. Tell me your theory again," said Lyn.

"Simply stated my theory is: Rheumatoid arthritis is caused by the inability of the adrenal glands to produce adequate corticosteroids."

"That sounds very straightforward."

"Yes, but where it becomes complicated is the manifold influences that directly affect the adrenal production of hormones. These are the issues that we must recognize and begin to control. If we can control the stress that we put on the adrenal glands, then we will not so easily fatigue them, and they will be able to produce more than adequate amounts of corticosteroids to keep you from the inflammatory pain caused by everyday friction."

"What are the factors then that make my adrenals tired?"

"The first and foremost is the consumption of sugar. Sugar has done more harm than any other one substance in our society. We all like to point at alcohol or cigarettes as agents of ill health—which they definitely are—but sugar escapes the anvil of condemnation because it is too near and dear to our hearts."

"You make it sound like we are in love with sugar," Lyn said.

"It's more than 'in love' with sugar. We are addicted to sugar. I do not say this lightly: we are a society that is in the throes of a real addiction. We adamantly deny it; we harshly criticize those who point it out to us; we attack verbally those that threaten our comfortable existence with this very insidious substance. We defend sugar's 'inability' to cause harm. We, as a society, reject the fact that sugar has addicting properties. Those that concede that it *might* be addictive are quick to emphasize its harmlessness even as it captures us in its claws of sweet ecstasy. Unfortunately, this attitude has permeated the mass of humanity to such an extent that change has become difficult to affect."

"But *everyone* eats sugar!"

"That's exactly what I mean. No one will believe that sugar is that damaging because everyone does it. Changing that belief is like trying to stop the ocean tides. But Lyn, if I can stop at least one drop of water in that ocean tide from traveling the current of destruction by sugar, then I have given that one drop a better life, a longer life, and a life that is filled with vibrant health."

"And I'm one of those drops."

"You are."

Karen could almost feel Lyn squaring her shoulders despite the invisibility that the phone lines could not overcome.

"Okay. Lay it on me. Tell me how sugar is destroying my life," Lyn said.

CHAPTER 7

Sugar Really Can Cause Rheumatoid Arthritis

"Anything that is a carbohydrate is converted to sugar," Karen began. "Not only are doughnuts, cakes, pies, cookies, and candies carbohydrates; but vegetables, fruits, cereals, breads, pasta, legumes, potatoes, and rice are also carbohydrates. Then we have nuts, seeds, milk, and cheese that are notable sources of carbohydrates. Carbohydrates are important. They are essential to life, but it is the speed at which the digestive system absorbs certain carbohydrates that becomes the issue."

"You mean some carbohydrates are absorbed faster than others?" Lyn asked.

"Yes, and the faster they are absorbed the more dangerous they become. I need to teach you a little bit more about the endocrine system. I've already told you some things about one of the sets of glands of the endocrine system—the adrenals—but you need to know more.

"There are several glands that make up the endocrine system. All of the glands of this system produce hormones. These hormones regulate myriads of bodily functions.

"The commanding officer of the endocrine system is called the pituitary gland. This little gland located at the base of your brain is under the directives of the hypothalamus. The hypothalamus is a part of your brain. The pituitary receives the command from the hypothalamus to keep blood sugars under control.

"As every good officer will do, the pituitary carries out his mission as directed. He constantly watches the blood sugar levels to make sure they stay in an acceptable range. The range is very narrow and if there is a deviation in where blood sugars are and where they should be, the pituitary immediately steps in and issues the orders to bring the sugars in line.

"Orders from the pituitary are carried by messengers called 'stimulating hormones.' These are the hormones that the pituitary itself secretes. The order is issued by the pituitary and the stimulating hormone carries the message to a gland called the pancreas. The pancreas is also a member of the endocrine system and thus under the command and control of the pituitary.

"The pancreas receives the written order from the hand of the messenger. Opening the message the pancreas reads, 'Release insulin in the following amount...'

"Insulin is a hormone that can grab the sugar molecules that are overrunning the system and disable them by converting them into fat. Please understand that the conversion of sugar into fat is absolutely critical to your survival."

Lyn interrupted, "But if the sugars are converted into fats, won't that make a person fat?"

"It most certainly can and often does! The converted sugars are called triglycerides and they create many problems besides obesity. Remember that thread I spun for you when I was talking about bile being made out of triglycerides? Too many triglycerides create problems for the heart. Now here's a new thread—triglycerides also make a person insulin resistant."

"Isn't insulin resistance related to diabetes?"

"Absolutely. And triglycerides and their effect on diabetes as well as the heart is another story for another day. The point that you must grasp now is that if the body is overrun with sugar, then insulin will turn the sugars into triglycerides to save you from a fatal condition called diabetic coma."

"So this really does have to do with diabetes."

"No, not yet. Eventually, if this reaction that I am explaining to you continues to happen over and over again, diabetes comes into the picture like an invited guest—but that isn't what's happening to you—yet. And *you* won't get to that place because today we are stopping this entire domino effect."

"Everything is related so closely to everything else, isn't it?" Lyn said with a touch of awe in her voice.

"Very much so. If a person can follow all the threads in the intricate tapestry of the human body, it's possible to solve the majority of our health problems. The study of this tapestry, the careful following of all the threads as they weave in and out of the pattern is what I have given myself to. I love this complicated discipline as it oftentimes results in being able to untangle what has always appeared as a snarl of threads that made no sense in the fabric. But on close inspection, the snarl is not a mess of tangled threads but a beautifully ordered pattern. We just didn't have the right pair of glasses to see it before. Seeing the threads clearly can result in cures that have not been possible."

"So you think there is a cure to rheumatoid arthritis?"

Karen answered without hesitation. "I do. The threads are laid out in a wondrously complex design, but their order is not hidden. Understanding the woven pattern *can* be done."

"If you are able to heal me of rheumatoid arthritis, I will be completely amazed."

Karen responded quietly, "I will heal you of nothing. I am just a simple tool in the hand of the Great Physician. He is the one that wove this incredible tapestry. He will be the one that heals you. And if God so uses me to be the instrument in his hand of healing, then I will stand with you, amazed at the great things that he has done."

Karen cleared her throat. Lyn could almost imagine that there were tears in Karen's eyes. If Lyn had been seated in Karen's office at that moment and not carrying on this conversation by telephone, she would have seen her suspicions confirmed. Karen *was* reaching for a tissue to wipe the moisture from her eyes before continuing.

"Lyn, you must comprehend this part about the sugar. It is paramount in your understanding of rheumatoid arthritis. If too much sugar enters your body too rapidly you are in danger of diabetic coma. It is the *rate of increase* in the blood sugar levels that is the critical piece here.

"The pituitary is supposed to keep your blood sugar levels in a very tight range. If large amounts of sugar are suddenly dumped into the bloodstream, then the pituitary will have to leap into action to stem the tide. Too much sugar will kill the brain."

Lyn interjected, "I don't get it, Karen. How can sugar possibly kill the brain? I've eaten lots of sugar. I love sugar! And my brain isn't dead!"

"No, your brain is certainly not dead," Karen laughed. "It's this pituitary action that prevents your murder by sugar. But you will pay, and pay heavily for making the pituitary constantly step in and save you from death time and time again."

Then Karen laughed again, "And, of course, you love sugar. Sugar is one of the major factors that has caused your rheumatoid arthritis. You have to be the carbohydrate queen to arrive at the throne of arthritis. I'll explain how you ascended to the throne!

"There are little fuel-burning factories within each and every human cell that must be fed a fuel to burn. These fuel-burning factories are called mitochondria. There are only two fuels that these factories accept and no others. The two fuels are fat and sugar.

"Every cell in the human body can burn either one of these fuels. If sugar is most available, the cells will burn sugar; if not, the cells will burn fat. It's a pretty neat dual-burning system.

"Now, I just said that all cells are dual-burners, but there is one exception. There is one system in the human body that cannot burn two fuels. It's a mono-burner system, only burning one type of fuel.

"The mono-burner in the human body is the central nervous system. This system includes your brain. Lyn, you have a fifty percent chance of getting this next question correct. As there are only two fuels, fat and sugar, which fuel does the central nervous system burn?"

Lyn hesitated before answering. She really wasn't sure. But Karen's emphasis had been on sugar, so she would take a stab at it. "Sugar."

"Correct! Sugar is the fuel of the central nervous system. Lyn, your brain runs on sugar! If you put too much sugar in your body too quickly you overload the brain with fuel.

"It's like flooding an engine. Think about it. Cars need gas to run. We give a car too much gas too quickly and we drown out the engine. The engine won't work! It is the same with sugar and the brain. If we flood the brain with too much sugar too quickly, the brain is drowned out and dies. It's called diabetic coma."

"All carbohydrates will be converted into blood sugar which is also known as glucose. The type of carbohydrate will dictate how much and how fast the blood glucose levels will rise. The simpler the carbohydrate, the faster we put sugar into the bloodstream. One of the worst carbohydrates we can consume is liquid sugars such as sodas or sweetened beverages, including fruit juice."

"Karen, I drink a lot of soda," Lyn admitted quietly.

"I know," Karen responded just as quietly. "You almost have to in order to arrive at the place where you are." Karen's voice was not condemnatory, simply acknowledging an already known fact.

"And fruit juice? Everyone knows that fruit juice is healthy."

"Fruit juice is *not* healthy. Unfortunately, the lie that it is healthy is perpetuated so continually that the vast majority of the public has believed it. The rapidity of the absorption of fruit juice is so incredibly high that it has joined forces with our other highly sugared foods and beverages to contribute to the disease states caused by sugar."

"But Karen . . ." Lyn began.

"Lyn, fruit has some wonderful properties as far as anti-oxidants, vitamins, minerals, and phytonutrients," Karen explained. "But these good things are adulterated when we concentrate the sugars in a piece of fruit into fruit juice. Fruit juice is an intensely sweet beverage. It causes an extremely rapid rise in our blood sugar that is very injurious to the endocrine system.

"Anytime we rapidly put large amounts of sugar into the bloodstream, the pituitary flies into a panic because soon Lyn will be dead from diabetic coma. Remember—it's flooding the engine. The pituitary releases huge amounts of a stimulating hormone to urge the pancreas to produce enough insulin to bring the soaring blood sugars down. But here is where the thread does a twist that most people miss. There is this law of nature that must be factored in: 'for every action in nature there is an equal and opposite reaction.'"

"I heard that in school dozens of times," Lyn said.

"And you should have, because it is a fact that we cannot dismiss in this apparent tangle in the weave. If your blood sugar levels are spiking, the amount of insulin released will be enough to bring down your blood sugar at the same rate as the spike. Now we will have rapidly falling blood sugars. This is called a crash.

"The crash creates a whole new set of problems. Just a few minutes ago your pituitary was worried about flooding the brain with too much sugar too quickly. Now the pituitary is faced with the opposite situation—not enough sugar to fuel the brain. If there is not enough sugar the brain will die. This is called insulin shock."

Lyn said, "Too bad that there is that 'equal and opposite' rule."

Karen replied, "The 'equal and opposite' rule is actually protective. The fault doesn't lie there. The fault is with the consumption of the sugary food or beverage. If a person didn't consume the sweets, then there would be no spike, and then there wouldn't be the subsequent crash."

"But sweets taste so good," Lyn moaned.

"I know, and yet we think it's just taste we like, but it's more than that. We've really set up an addictive cycle. When the blood sugars come crashing down, we'll have but a short time before we enter insulin shock. The pituitary sees this problem and steps in to correct the situation. In the meantime, the brain has implemented protective measures also. Both are working for the same goal: get sugar into the bloodstream to fuel the central nervous system.

"First, I'll tell you what the brain will do. The brain simultaneously works in two ways. It will tell you in very strong language that you are hungry, and not just hungry for a boiled egg or a piece of chicken. You want a carbohydrate—in fact the simpler the carbohydrate the better. Actually, if that carbohydrate could be sweet we'll have faster results. Remember that carbohydrates are converted into blood glucose very easily and quickly. If the carbohydrate is a sweet, then the blood sugar levels will be replenished very rapidly—even in seconds.

"When I said that you 'want' a carbohydrate, I didn't state it strongly enough. Even 'crave' is not adequate to describe the immense desire, an all-consuming thought that you *must* have something sweet to eat and you must have it *now*!

"We have an emergency situation because your body is careening toward death because there are insufficient amounts of sugar to fuel your brain. Without that sugar, the life-communicating neurotransmitters cannot be made."

"Whoa. What are neurotransmitters?" Lyn asked.

"Neurotransmitters close the electrical circuit that allows the brain to communicate with the entire body. Most people don't realize that the brain sends tiny electrical voltages down wires called neural fibers. No one neural fiber is connected to another neural fiber. They are all short pieces of 'wire' that don't touch one another. There is a space between the ends of the wires called a synapse. These spaces are gaps between the neural fibers. If that gap is not bridged by a conductive material then the electricity cannot traverse the gap and the message dies on the wire."

"Wow, so the body is like an electrical circuit," Lyn said.

"It is without a doubt," Karen replied. "The conductive material that has to fill the synaptic gap must be made by cells located at the ends of the neural fibers. The conductive substances that are produced by these cells are called neurotransmitters."

Karen paused. "Lyn, these cells have to have some sort of fuel to burn to be able to have the energy to produce the neurotransmitters."

"And that fuel is sugar," Lyn filled in. "I'm starting to get it."

"If the brain does not have enough sugar, the neurotransmitters cannot be made. The messages will not reach the intended source and death will result. Lyn, did you know that for every beat of your heart the brain has sent an electrical message to tell it to beat?"

"I never really thought about it before, but I guess I somehow knew it," Lyn answered.

"For every beat of the heart, for every breath that we take, for every drop of blood that the kidneys and the liver filter, for every bodily function that happens—the brain has sent an electrical message to make it happen. Without sugar, we will cease to exist."

"That almost makes me think that we should be eating sugary things to keep the brain running," Lyn said.

Karen sighed. "That is an excuse that many people use. They actually believe that consuming large amounts of sugar is good for them or at least okay for that very reason—brain fuel. The acceptance and embracing of sugar as a harmless and even beneficial food is a big mistake. It means trouble, Trouble, TROUBLE!"

"Do you ever get frustrated because the whole world is crazy about sugar?"

There was a long pause before Lyn heard Karen's voice in reply. "Frustration is not what I feel. It's more like a deep sadness for all the people who will live less than full lives. For all the people who will die miserable deaths. For all the people who will perish years sooner than was necessary. Lyn, what I do feel is that I'm a fish swimming upstream against the current of society. All society, even the health industry, embraces sugar."

"Sugar is everywhere," Lyn agreed. "At home, in the office—wherever I turn there are cookies, cakes, pies, doughnuts, and candy."

"Yes," Karen replied. "It's even in the doctors' offices and hospitals. For years, doctors have handed out suckers to children to comfort them from the trauma of being at their office. Recently, doctors' offices have switched to giving out stickers instead of candy, but they still have the sweets in the break room for themselves and their employees. The hospitals serve desserts on the trays that are delivered to a patient's room, and even the hospital dieticians say sugar is okay in reasonable quantities or recommend an artificial sweetener, which is worse than sugar."

"Artificial sweeteners are worse than sugar?" Lyn asked incredulously.

"Yes. And I'll tell you why, but first I have to finish telling you how the endocrine system responds to sugar and how that has helped create your rheumatoid arthritis. We've veered off the main subject onto a side path."

"Sorry about that, but there is just so much I want to know."

Karen laughed. "I could lecture for days and years on these topics because I want people like you to know these things. But for now and the sake of your phone bill I'll try to keep the explanation to a reasonable length.

"Back to the massive problem that the endocrine system is facing: we are running out of fuel for the brain and spiraling faster and faster toward insulin shock. All life is about to cease. The brain has given you the very strong message to eat sugar so that we can stop the death run. In the meantime, while you are debating whether to fulfill the craving that you suddenly have, the brain institutes other measures to stave off the eventual cessation of life. I call it 'brain triage.'"

"I heard the term 'triage' while I was training in the Army. It means to allocate aid on the basis of need," Lyn said.

"Nice job! Most people don't know what that word means," Karen said. "And you are absolutely correct. In our case, the brain uses triage to determine where it will spend what little sugar it has. The brain has many systems to run. As the fuel resources are running low, the brain gets pretty picky on which functions will be fueled and which functions will fall by the wayside.

"The brain will choose to operate the part of the central nervous system that controls life-support. That means the brain will use what little sugar it has to run the heart, lungs, kidneys, liver, and other essential operations for existence. All other functions of the central nervous system will be neglected.

"These neglected functions are things like emotional control, memory, cognitive thought, and visual acuity. The brain will not waste what precious little fuel it has on things that are superfluous to life-support.

"Therefore, you will find when you have a sugar crash that you are no longer as 'happy' as you were a few moments before. In fact, you are downright ornery. It's called a mood swing. I call it 'Dr. Jekyll and Mr. Hyde behavior.' One moment you are pleasant and reasonable, the next moment you're not! If you have a strong-willed type of personality you'll become easily angered. If you have the peace-maker type of personality you'll break down in a heap of tears. You are not able to make enough neurotransmitters to maintain emotional control because the brain will not allow that waste of fuel.

"Another frittering away of fuel is the futile production of the neurotransmitters that allow you to access your memory cells. The real priority is to keep your heart beating—not remember what you were about to say. So you'll find yourself telling someone a story or explaining a procedure, and they interrupt you to say something. You start to pick up where you left off, but suddenly you can't remember what you were about to say. You try your best to recall, but you come up blank.

"Or you will be in your kitchen doing something and you think to yourself, 'Oh those scissors are in the bedroom. I need those so I'll go get them.' You walk to the bedroom which may only be a few paces away. You arrive in the bedroom and ...you can't remember what you came into the bedroom for. You remember that you were going to retrieve something, but you can't remember what. You stand there like a dunce thinking that you have the early onset of Alzheimer's! But the real problem is that you are not making the neurotransmitters to retrieve the information you need."

Lyn said, "You're describing what happens to me all the time."

"There's more," Karen said. "Without sufficient fuel to make the neurotransmitters, your thinking becomes impaired. You will have difficulty in putting sentences together; you will turn words around in your sentence; you will not be able to deal with numbers very well. I call it cognitive fuzziness or brain fog. It's not severe enough to earn a diagnosis—we just know that we aren't thinking as sharply and clearly as just a little while ago."

Karen decided to give Lyn a true-life illustration. "A few years ago, I was visiting one of our parishioners who had had surgery. He was in our local hospital on the medical-surgery ward. I was seated in his room and the door to the hallway was open. As we were visiting, a nurse pushing a gurney with a patient still groggy from surgery stopped right outside the door. Another nurse was approaching from the opposite direction. The nurse pushing the gurney said to the approaching nurse, 'Would you help me move the room into the bed?' The other nurse replied in the affirmative without even blinking an eye, and they went down the hall together. Of course, we all knew that the woman had meant to say, 'Would you help me move the bed into the room?' This happens so frequently that people don't even comment on it—if they notice it at all!

"I sat there knowing that the nurse was in a low blood sugar crash—and the obvious reason was that she had recently consumed something that was sweet. I hoped that she wouldn't get so fuddle-brained that she would make a mistake with the man's IV's and give him something that he shouldn't have. I even thought about following the nurse down the hall and recommending that she get something to eat to stop her crash, but decided that my advice would not be well received. So I kept my seat and continued to visit as if I had heard nothing.

"I myself used to feel like this all the time, before I became a nutritionist and learned so much, and *applied* what I learned. I never knew the freedom of feeling cognitively succinct on a continual basis until I ditched the sugars out of my life."

"*You* used to eat sugars?" Lyn asked.

"Oh yes, because I didn't know better. Actually, as a child I lived off cinnamon toast—the quick kind where it's a piece of white bread, buttered, sprinkled liberally with white sugar, dusted with cinnamon, and then toasted. Heavily sugared ice tea would complete my meal.

"It resulted in my having Grave's disease at the age of seventeen and a subsequent almost-total thyroidectomy. That's another subject I would love to cover: thyroid disorders, their supposed causes, the real cause, and the solution—which is not surgery! But as that doesn't apply to you, we'll skip that for today."

"Good grief, you know a bunch about a lot of health problems," Lyn said.

"I've been practicing for almost two decades. A person learns a lot during that amount of time. But back to the effects of sugar!

"There are other signs of low blood sugar such as visual changes—you just don't see as well as you did before. It's temporary, but a nuisance. You can feel shaky, dizzy, and if the crash is especially bad a person can even pass out.

"These crashes are a huge strain on the endocrine system. First the system had to compensate for a spike in blood sugars—and now the system must compensate for the crash in sugars that was caused by the spike!

"You see, while the brain is trying to cope by using triage, your blood sugar is still falling. Once insulin is released, we cannot tell it to stop its work. We can tell the pancreas to stop secreting insulin, which the pituitary will certainly do. But what about all that insulin that is rounding up the sugars like prisoners and herding them away into fat cells?"

"What?" Lyn interjected. "Fat cells?"

"Insulin converts sugars into fats, which are stored in our adipose tissue," Karen responded.

"Adipose tissue?"

"Yes. Adipose tissue is just a fancy way to say 'fat cells.' Bottom line—sugar is converted into fat and a person gets fat!"

"Oh, boy," Lyn sighed.

Karen pushed on. So much to say and it had to be communicated well so that Lyn would understand.

"Lyn, if a person does not eat when the brain is shouting the message 'Hey, we're dying here. We need sugar. Please eat!' then another domino falls. And this domino is the one that has caused your rheumatoid arthritis or at the very least has been a major player.

"This is the information I've been waiting to hear," Lyn said.

"There is this very narrow window of time when you absolutely must eat to prevent insulin shock. The narrowness of the window depends on the intensity and amount of the sweet that was just consumed. The more sugar the narrower your window. If you do not eat in those few minutes—and normally it is less than thirty minutes after a sweet has been consumed—although it can be as short as one minute—your brain will begin Plan B.

"Plan A was: Brain, get the woman to eat so that we can stop the plunge into insulin shock. Do that by putting a craving in her head for sweets. But this plan didn't work. You didn't eat in the prescribed time. Now the body must move to Plan B. That is: Is there any sugar *stored* in the body that we can access?

"There is only one solution to stop insulin shock. We must put sugar in the bloodstream so the brain can function. If you don't eat it, then we must find another way to get sugar. Plan B is another way. There is also a Plan C—and that is the last straw—there is no other plan after that. But it is Plan B that has gotten you into trouble with rheumatoid arthritis.

"Sugar is *not* normally stored in the human body. As I told you before, it is converted into fat tucked away into little rolls of flesh on our bodies—and I need to mention here that it is also stored in the blood itself as triglycerides. Don't let this information distract you, but it's another thread in the pattern that leads us to the diabetes as well as heart disease piece of fabric. Suffice it to say right now: we convert sugars to fats.

"But despite this fact, the body has squirreled away some sugar just in case a situation like this occurs, as the brain can't burn fat as a fuel. The body has two hidden sources of sugar kept in case of dire need. Well, this is one of those times. By now, you are just minutes from entering the fog of insulin shock and the brain is insisting that emergency measures be taken."

"So where are these hidden troves of sugar?" Lyn asked.

"The first is found in the muscle tissue. The sugar is called muscle glycogen. There is enough fuel there to keep the brain in operation for a few minutes."

"That's not very long."

"You're right. It's not very long at all. That's why we will need to target the second cache of sugar. It's found in the liver. It's also called glycogen. There is enough liver glycogen to fuel the brain for several hours. So that becomes the answer. Release the liver glycogen!

"But here's the catch: glycogen will not just flow out of the liver. It must be *told* to come out—and hormones do the telling. Would you like to guess the name of the hormone that is responsible for delivering the order to the liver to release glycogen?"

"I'm almost afraid to find out. No guessing. Just tell me," Lyn answered.

Karen's voice was flat as she said, "Adrenalin."

"This is the adrenalin that is made in the adrenal glands?"

"None other," Karen responded. It was time to drive the point home. "Lyn, you make the adrenal glands jump through hoops in producing these large amounts of adrenalin to respond to sugar emergencies. Over time, the adrenals become fatigued. Not only will they not produce adequate amounts of adrenalin which give you zippety-do-dah when you want it, but *they will be unable to produce the amount of corticosteroids necessary to keep you from the pain of everyday friction.*"

"And the lack of these corticosteroids has caused my rheumatoid arthritis?"

"Yes, that's my theory. And I would like to prove that theory to you by having you eliminate sugar as well as the other adrenal stressors. If your rheumatoid arthritis is cured, then we will know that my theory is correct."

"So 'no sweets' will be a part of 'the lists.'"

"Yes, ma'am," Karen responded. "It is. As well as no fruit juice and no fruit. Eventually you will get to eat fruit again, once you're well—but we can't even afford this during the healing process."

"Fruit has tons of nutrients," Lyn said somewhat defensively.

"You're right. Fruit does. It also has large amounts of naturally occurring sugar which is enough to tip you over the edge into endocrine stress. Don't worry about missing the nutrients as you'll be getting them in even larger quantities in your vegetables, which I will be requiring you to eat once we settle down the ulcerative colitis."

"But what vegetable could replace an orange? Everyone knows that oranges are our best source of vitamin C."

"Actually, oranges are not our best source. The average orange has seventy milligrams of vitamin C. One cup of chopped red sweet pepper has two hundred thirty-two milligrams of vitamin C. As a fact, our vegetables are more nutrient-dense than our fruits. *And* vegetables come with significantly less sugar."

Lyn needed a moment to absorb this. Taking someone's sweets away was a major shock. But then fruit juice and fruit! She was not sure she really could stay away from these things. But the thought flashed through Lyn's head—do I want to stay locked in this prison of pain? No! Determination flooded through Lyn's being.

"Karen, I will do it."

"Bravo, Lyn, bravo!"

"Karen, before you go on—my curiosity is getting the better of me—what happens if I use up all my stored glycogen and I still haven't eaten? People go on fasts for days and they don't die of insulin shock."

"Ah. Then the body moves to the final attempt to stave off death. Plan C—otherwise known as ketosis."

"I've heard of diets that use ketosis as a means to lose weight."

"Yes. And they are not wise to implement. Ketosis is a very difficult and dangerous state for the body to be in. When the glycogen stores are exhausted, and for whatever reason you are not ingesting any carbohydrates to fuel the brain, then the body is forced to convert a protein into a sugar."

"If the body can convert a protein into a sugar, can it also convert a fat into a sugar?" Lyn asked.

"I wish. But a conversion of fat into sugar is not possible."

Karen continued, "The liver does the work of converting the proteins into sugar. The protein molecules are taken from your muscle tissue. This conversion is called deaminization. After a time this process becomes a strain on the liver as well as a strain on the kidneys. In fact, it's a stress on the whole body. The reason is that during deaminization there is a byproduct that is released into the blood. Ammonia."

"Ammonia," Lyn said. "That's poisonous."

"Very much so. That's why the kidneys leap into action to filter the ammonia out of the bloodstream. The increased filtering action of the kidneys oftentimes lead to kidney stones as they pull out not only the ammonia but larger amounts of water soluble nutrients—the major one being calcium. That's why it's common to develop kidney stones while on these types of ketosis diets. This is another path that I won't travel with you today as it isn't applicable to your situation."

"So ketosis is Plan C," Lyn mused.

"Yep. I will never recommend a plan for healing that involves ketosis. It's just way too harmful to the body. Now that I've hopefully satisfied your curiosity about the third and last way that the body saves you from insulin shock, I need to tickle your ears with some other data of which you need to be apprised, if we are going to heal you of rheumatoid arthritis."

8

CHAPTER 8

Other Little Nasties That Wear Out the Adrenals

Karen took a drink of water. The time and effort it took to educate a client never seemed an onerous chore to her. But it was certainly work. A labor of love she thought to herself. If I can help just one person get better, then it's all worth it.

"Lyn, you now understand how sugar impacts the adrenal system. It puts such a heavy load on the two adrenal glands that it's only a matter of time before they become worn out."

"I understand," Lyn replied.

"There are several other things that also fatigue the adrenals to the point that they are unable to make adequate corticosteroids to keep you out of pain. After sugar, the next biggest aggravator is caffeine."

"So now you're going to pick on my soda," Lyn sighed.

"And your coffee and tea," Karen responded. "Caffeine directly stimulates the adrenals to produce more adrenalin. Caffeine is a whip to those glands, forcing them to work harder. That's why people drink caffeinated beverages or take caffeine pills. They get an adrenalin rush from them.

"Adrenalin is our 'feel-good' hormone. It gives us a sense of well-being. It gives us zest, motivation, zippety-do-dah—the ability to live life in full color versus black-and-white. Everybody wants to feel this way. If we don't feel this way we sink into depression."

"You're kidding. Adrenalin has something to do with depression?" Lyn asked.

"It has everything to do with depression. Adrenalin is a neurotransmitter despite its being made in the endocrine system. It is actually made of the hormones epinephrine and norepinephrine—the two most powerful neurotransmitters that we have. But this is another one of those threads that I will not follow for you today. I only explain the details of those designs with my clients that suffer with depression and anxiety."

"Wow," Lyn said. "There is so much to know. I want to learn as much as I can."

"Me, too," Karen responded.

"What? You already know this stuff!" Lyn said.

"I only know small bits and pieces. The vastness of the knowledge is so great that if I study for a lifetime, I'll never learn it all. I have such an insatiable desire to learn. I've actually asked God to give me three or four lifetimes in the space of my one. I want to understand as much information as I can in order to use that knowledge to accomplish many things. One of my greatest passions is to apply what I learn in a practical way so that people's lives are changed for the better. Knowledge is one thing, but the application of that knowledge is another. That's my goal—application of knowledge."

"Well, I think you are achieving it. You certainly seem to be taking a lot of scientific principles and applying them to get me well," Lyn replied. Then she added, "If I really do get well."

"That is to be seen. But I can tell you this, Lyn, you are not the first person with whom I have worked that has ulcerative colitis and rheumatoid arthritis. I've had wonderful results with others. I don't believe that you'll be any different. I'm expecting that you'll heal completely."

"I hope so, I really hope so."

"Hope will have nothing to do with it. It'll be a matter of cells healing or not healing. If we can learn what the cause is and correct the aberrant behavior, then healing will take place. It's a simple matter of cause and effect."

Then Karen added, "My heart is with yours, Lyn. I also hope that the knowledge and wisdom that I have will be the answer. And in your situation, it should be. But then there are always curve balls."

"Curve balls?"

Karen laughed. "Yes. Twists and turns that are totally unexpected. Actually, I like curve balls. It makes my life interesting and fun! Then I get to run down paths that lead me to unexpected places, and I find that fascinating."

"Well, I hope I don't throw you any curve balls," Lyn stated. "I just want to get well."

"Don't worry, so far I haven't seen anything in your condition that is an enigma, and although I do love a good mystery, you are pretty easy to solve. So, no, I'm not expecting any curve balls from you."

"Good."

"Alright, back on topic—we were talking about caffeine being one of the little cruel fellows that stresses the adrenal glands, making the adrenals unable to produce enough of the anti-inflammatory hormones called corticosteroids."

"I'm with you."

Karen could almost see Lyn scribbling away as she took notes. "Caffeine causes the endocrine system to fly into quite a fit because caffeine is regarded as unfriendly by the body. Unfriendly substances are potentially dangerous, and the body will be anxious to be rid of them. So we have to have a mechanism to clean them out of the bloodstream.

"That mechanism is found in the action of the liver and the kidneys. These organs are constantly filtering the bloodstream to remove toxins such as caffeine. There are other offending substances, but I won't denounce them quite yet.

"The problem is that the brain isn't satisfied with the filtering action of the liver and kidneys when these perpetrators enter the bloodstream. The brain demands that the filtering process be speeded to facilitate the rapid removal of these unwanted substances. However, the speed of filtration is not dependent on the liver and kidneys. These organs are static. They do not actively reach out into the bloodstream and grab the mean little goons faster. They can only filter as fast as the blood flows through them.

"Therefore, if we want to increase the speed of filtration, we must increase the speed of the blood flowing through these organs. If we could raise the blood pressure, we will increase the speed of the blood. The rise in blood pressure does not have to be substantial, even a small increase will accomplish the mission."

"You explained this to me before when we were talking about medications. It's the garden hose illustration, isn't it?"

"It is. Remember that we have to constrict the blood vessels to increase blood pressure."

"And adrenalin is the hormone that accomplishes this," Lyn finished.

"Good! Now, I want you to absorb and remember this data. If you do, it will help you face the lists."

"Oh, yeah," Lyn shivered. "The lists."

Karen smiled at Lyn's affected dread. "So here's the bottom line: if you take caffeine into your body you will have an adrenal response. The more caffeine, the more adrenalin. And the more adrenalin you produce above and beyond what is considered maintenance amounts, the faster you fatigue those glands."

"So caffeine is on the lists," Lyn said.

"Yes. In fact, every adrenal stressor that we can possibly remove from your life will be on that list."

Karen continued. "Now you understand why people drink caffeinated beverages. The caffeine causes an adrenal rush. Adrenalin is our feel-good, think bright, let's rip-roar hormone. The more we have of this the better we feel."

"So the caffeine in my soda is making my rheumatoid arthritis worse," Lyn thought out loud.

"Making it worse and more than that—actually causing the rheumatoid arthritis." Karen waited just a short moment before adding, "And decaffeinated products are harmful in the same way."

"Wait a minute. Decaffeinated products don't have any caffeine!" Lyn protested.

"Actually they do. They have significantly less caffeine than the original product, but there is not a process that can remove *all* the caffeine. Decaffeinated products still have caffeine."

"But if they have less caffeine, it stands to reason that they would cause less harm."

"Correct. However, the decaffeination process[5] itself leaves several harsh chemical residues that stimulate the adrenals to speed the filtration process by causing vasoconstriction.

"If you doubt what I say, consider the people who consume decaffeinated beverages such as coffee. They know that their decaf coffee gives them a pick-me-up, and will even keep them awake at night if they drink it too late in the evening. Only adrenalin can cause this type of action. The decaffeinated beverage has triggered the adrenals."

"Okay, okay. So no decaf."

"Lyn, I have to break the news to you that there are other things that do the very same thing as caffeine and decaffeinated products—some at lower levels, some at higher levels."

---

5   See appendix for further remarks and references.

There was a sigh on the other end of the phone line but no response. Karen continued, "The mechanism of action is the same for all of them. They are whips to the adrenal glands. They force an already fully functioning gland to function at even higher levels. This sustained demand eventually wears the glands to the point that they can no longer function at levels that will provide you sufficient adrenalin—or sufficient corticosteroids."

"So then I feel pain because I don't have enough grease between my joints."

"You got it."

"What are the other things besides caffeine that are wreaking havoc on my adrenals?" Lyn asked.

"The next is artificial sweeteners."

"Don't tell me that! I already figured you were going to take sugar away from me, so I had mentally planned on using artificial sweeteners," Lyn groaned.

"Sorry." Karen couldn't keep the grin from her face. Even if Lyn was sitting across from her, she would still have grinned. Lyn was an enjoyable client. It was fun to talk to someone who was so sharp and had a sense of humor.

Lyn made a try for a least some of the artificial sweeteners. "Well, certainly that doesn't include the natural-artificial sweeteners, does it?"

"Oxymorons," Karen said. "They're always interesting. Doesn't 'artificial' cancel out 'natural?' I didn't make up the term 'natural-artificial sweeteners,' but unfortunately I have to repeat it often. Oh well."

"What about the sugar alcohols, and, and . . ." Lyn was searching for the word.

"Stevia—the 'sweet leaf,'" Karen supplied for her.

"Yeah," Lyn confirmed. "Are they okay?"

"No. They are not okay. They also stress the body in the same way as caffeine. They cause an adrenal response. Have you ever thought about the reason that people consume artificially sweetened products? They get a kick from them. Whether it's a power bar sweetened with a natural-artificial substance or a diet soda sweetened with aspartame, they all give the eater a boost—and this includes those products that are caffeine-free."

"But Karen, some people should be drinking diet sodas because they need to lose weight."

Karen hooted with laughter. "Oh, Lyn, diet sodas don't help anyone lose weight. They actually cause people to gain weight! The increased adrenal response includes an amplified production of aldosterone—another adrenal hormone. Aldosterone tells the kidneys to retain salt. Salt draws water to itself. And the person gains weight because their body holds water."

"It's another thread," Lyn said with a touch of surprise.

"Yep. So many threads to follow. But despite the complexity of the pattern we will still be able to comprehend enough that we can affect positive change—even healing. For you, Lyn, and for today, artificial sweeteners will be added to your list."

"I've got it down. What's next?"

"There is a list of other little terrors that I will rattle off but not go into detail about them because you are not currently consuming any of them, but just be aware that these guys cause the same type of stress on the adrenals: licorice, ephedra which is also called ma-huang, ephedrine, pseudoephedrine, gotu kola, dong quai, and even black cohosh.

"And now two more to add to this list—the first is perfume and then if that doesn't blow your socks off, the next one will. But first, I'll explain perfumes and fragrances.

"It's the same reaction that happens in the human body as with any of the other substances that I have already mentioned. The liver and the kidneys have to filter faster to clean out the offensive fragrance. To do this, adrenalin must be released to facilitate vasoconstriction. Perfumes cause an adrenal response."

"Even natural fragrances like essential oils?" Lyn asked.

"Even the essential oils. Aroma therapy is not all that it's cracked up to be."

"Karen, you're flying in the face of some established natural practices. Aroma therapy is touted everywhere as being healthy."

"I know." This time it was Karen's turn to sigh. "But just because it's proclaimed as a health measure, doesn't mean that it is. Aroma therapy works because it is a whip to the endocrine system. The subsequent release of hormones *does* make a person feel better. But a person can drink a soda or a cup of coffee, smoke a cigarette, or take a diet pill—which will have some form of stimulant in it—and they will *feel* better. But using all these things is like taking a bull whip to the adrenals, demanding more production than they are currently able to do.

"Imagine you have two horses that are pulling a heavily loaded wagon. You work these creatures hard. You don't feed them particularly well, but at least you let them sleep a little—usually six to seven hours a day before you demand that they work again. You know that it's really not enough rest for them, but you have so much work for them to do that you decide not to allow them any more.

"After a time of carrying this grueling work load, you are very disappointed that the horses aren't moving as quickly. In fact, they slow to such an extent that they are not getting all the work done. You cluck and talk to the horses, but they move no faster. You decide that it's time for the whip. Whips on horses are very effective. After a few lashes on the backs of those animals, they are on the move again, trotting along at a good pace.

"'There,' you say to yourself, 'they only needed a little "motivation."' Of course, you know that your motivation was a bit cruel, but at least it worked. As the days and weeks go by, you have to continue to apply the whips to keep those horses moving. In fact, you note that the whip is required more often and sometimes you have to be downright merciless as you beat the tar out of the animals to make them move."

"My adrenal glands are those horses, aren't they?" Lyn asked.

"Yes, and the whips are sugar, caffeine, artificial sweeteners, that list of other stimulants I gave you, *and* fragrances," Karen replied. "Without knowing it, you have been using whips to make the adrenals function at a higher level. But beating the glands will not heal them. In fact, they only become less functional. The way to heal them is to stop whipping them, let them rest, and feed them the right food. Then they will recover and be able to function fully for you—without the use of whips."

"Karen, are you sure that *all* fragrances have this effect?"

"Let me put it this way, Lyn. When a person breathes in a perfume or fragrance they will note a difference in the way they feel. Mostly, they will have a sense of well-being. Adrenalin is the hormone that gives us a sense of well-being. Remember that adrenalin is composed of our two most powerful neurotransmitters."

"Is that how an aphrodisiac works?"

"Yes. Libido or sexual desire is controlled by the hormones estrogen and testosterone—not adrenalin. But when adrenalin is released, every other hormone that the endocrine system makes is also released. The endocrine system works as a family of glands. When one family member is stressed and overworking—all of the family is stressed and overworks.

"That's why these adrenal stressors that I have been describing to you should really be called endocrine system stressors. The entire endocrine system becomes tired which results in low thyroid function, poor sleep habits, irregular and painful menstrual cycles, and more. It's way too much to cover with you now, Lyn, but suffice it to say that I have begun to reveal only the tip of the iceberg."

"Karen, can a person even live in this world without exposure to perfumes?"

"We can at least live without twenty-four-hour-a-day-seven-day-a-week exposure to fragrances. Your home and the lack of fragrances on your body can be a safe haven. That alone will minimize your exposure to a great degree, and thus minimize the stress on the adrenals."

"Does that mean I can't even burn scented candles?"

"It does. I'll be very specific when we move to the lists. But now I have to drop the bombshell on you."

Lyn's voice was wry as she replied, "As if you haven't already dropped several."

CHAPTER 9

The Little Nasty That Has Become a Big Nasty Because It Is So Misunderstood

"If you thought that I was flying in the face of the proponents of aroma therapy, you will find that I am now going to challenge a vastly larger bastion of the health industry. The people who are fully endorsing of this principle of health include not only doctors, but chiropractors, and every other health profession out there. Before I announce this startling concept, I must preface it by telling you that the abstention from this practice is only temporary. Once you are healed of your rheumatoid arthritis, you will find me tolerant of and in most cases a supporter of this practice."

"You really have me incredibly curious. What is it that's so earth-shattering?"

"Exercise."

The bomb impacted and Karen waited for Lyn's initial shock to pass. Lyn's words came out as a splutter, "But my doctor told me that I *need* to exercise to help my rheumatoid arthritis. I've been forcing myself to walk despite the pain because it's supposed to *help* me!"

"The exercise has only kept you locked in the vicious jaws of your arthritis."

"But ...but how?"

"The hormone that has to be produced to get your body in motion and to keep your body in motion is adrenalin." Karen waited for this to sink in. "Exercise requires tremendous adrenalin production. A person simply cannot maintain exercise without it."

"But when I am walking and exercising, I really do feel less pain!" Lyn objected.

"My point exactly," Karen calmly replied. "Lyn, think for a moment. If you are making more adrenalin to sustain your exercise, then you have to make accompanying amounts of corticosteroid at the very same time. These hormones are made in the *same* glands."

There was a long silence. In a barely audible voice Karen heard Lyn murmur, "If I make more corticosteroid because I'm making more adrenalin, my inflammation is less."

Karen finished for her. "And the exercise is a whip, just like any other. We have not helped the glands to heal; we have just put another stress on them." Karen paused before continuing. This was a lot to take in. "You can drink soda and it will give you the same result as the exercise—less pain and more energy—but it's only for a very short time. Any whip—whether soda, coffee, perfume, artificial sweeteners, or exercise will give you an adrenal response that is erroneously viewed as positive. That's why people do these things. They aren't consciously thinking, 'I'll have a cup of coffee or I'll exercise to beat my adrenals into action.' They simply know that somehow they feel better."

"I've been self-medicating all along," Lyn said. "I've been using adrenal whips, never knowing that I've been causing more harm than good." There was urgency in her next words, "Karen, we've got to get this information known! There are so many people who are under the wrong perception."

Karen didn't respond right away. The familiar burden weighed her down once again. So many people. So many people hurting who didn't have to hurt. For the thousandth time, she resolved to try to help them somehow.

"Karen, are you there?" Lyn's voice came through the receiver loudly.

"Yes, I'm here." Karen responded. "I'm sorry, Lyn, I was just thinking about what you said. Yes, we need to get the message out. I'm working as hard as I can to do just that."

Returning to the subject at hand Karen said, "You can now see why you felt better while you were actually *doing* the exercise—when your body was in motion. But if you recall accurately, you'll realize after the exercise was completed that you hurt just as much, and in fact, more than you had hurt before your exercise."

"I had always thought my increased pain was because I didn't exercise enough," Lyn said.

"It's a logical conclusion to make because a person hears so much about the wonderful benefits of exercise, specifically the catabolic and anabolic states of metabolic degeneration and regeneration. So we strictly attribute our pain to these processes."

"Wait. Say that again."

"What I mean to tell you is this: You thought your aches and pains were normal muscle soreness."

"Yes, I did."

"*Your* pain incurred by exercise is not normal muscle soreness. You rubbed the joints together more rapidly and more often which created more friction. The additional friction resulted in more heat. The increased heat without sufficient corticosteroid to negate its effects damaged your tissue creating inflammation and pain. The more a person moves, Lyn, the more friction occurs."

"I totally understand. The added movement means that I would need extra corticosteroid to compensate, but my problem is that I don't make enough corticosteroid to begin with so I actually made things worse."

"Yes," Karen said.

"But I still have a question about exercise. It's supposed to be good for your heart. A person hears that everywhere. How can my heart stay healthy without exercise?"

Karen smiled. So much to teach. It was a good thing that she enjoyed it. "Your heart is a muscle like any other. When we work a muscle it will become stronger. That's a result of sheer necessity. If we put more load on a certain muscle, it needs to grow stronger to carry that load. Simple cause and effect. Therefore, if we exercise the heart muscle by increasing the load then the heart will grow stronger."

"And exercise increases the workload on the heart," Lyn concluded.

"Yes. But how does exercise increase the load on the heart?" Karen asked.

Lyn hesitated. She had not thought about it before. "Well, I suppose by beating harder and more frequently."

Karen persisted, "Yes, but what mechanism makes the heart beat harder and more frequently?"

Lyn shook her head. She really didn't know. "I'm not sure," she finally said.

"Don't feel bad for not knowing. Most people don't ever think it through. If a person is exercising they use more oxygen. Oxygen is absolutely essential to muscle tissue. Without it, fuels cannot be burned. When a fat or sugar—the two fuels about which I already taught you—are burned or metabolized with the aid of oxygen we give the muscle cells the energy to do the work.

"If we are exercising, the work increases. Therefore the energy needs increase and we need more oxygen. Now the problem is getting the oxygen to the muscle cells more quickly. Enter the heart.

"The heart is responsible for pushing the blood to the needed muscles. It is a pump forcing this life-giving liquid that carries oxygen to the places where it is needed. If you are using muscles at an accelerated rate then the oxygen requirements increase dramatically. The heart pumps harder and more frequently to keep up with the demand.

"Now, here is the part that most people don't realize. What makes the heart beat harder and faster?" Karen did not wait for Lyn to answer. "Adrenalin, Lyn, adrenalin. Remember that adrenalin is a powerful vasoconstrictor. It causes the blood vessels to narrow in order to increase the blood pressure. Remember the garden hose illustration?"

"I do. If we constrict the space that the same amount of liquid has to flow through, it increases the speed at which the liquid travels," Lyn responded.

"Excellent! So now let's connect the dots. If the blood is traveling at higher speeds due to increased pressure, the heart has to work harder. Therefore, the heart will deliver oxygen to the needed areas in a timely fashion. If we force the heart to work harder, we are exercising the heart muscle." Karen paused before delivering the conclusion. She needed to make sure that Lyn understood this completely. "*A release of adrenalin, from whatever cause, will exercise the heart.*"

There was silence on Lyn's end of the phone. Finally she spoke, "You mean that if I have a cup of coffee or drink a soda then I'm exercising my heart?"

"Yes. People who have more than the average adrenalin production due to whatever reason—stress, caffeine, sugar intake or any other adrenal stressor—they are exercising their heart. They don't need to run or walk on the treadmill for cardiovascular health. Exercise will help in the strengthening of other muscles like leg or arm muscles—but the cardiovascular system is covered more than adequately."

"If people knew this they would quit exercising and increase their soda drinking," Lyn said incredulously.

"But if they used the soda for the adrenalin stimulation they would only wear out the glands more quickly and end up with adrenal fatigue—just like you. No, the answer is not to exercise the heart by using stimulants; the point is that stimulants *do* exercise the heart. *Adrenalin* does exercise the heart, resulting in strengthening that muscle. I need to add here—and this is very important—that *too much* adrenalin strains the heart muscle by adding *too much* work.

"The beginning and the end of all this, Lyn, is that you have been exercising your heart with every adrenal release that you have forced—and you have been doing it for years. Your cardiovascular health is good. You will not have to worry about the lack of exercise resulting in poor heart health. Good grief, woman, you're an adrenalin machine. That's how you got in this predicament in the first place."

"Karen, do you think that most people are adrenalin machines?"

"No, I don't. The majority of people do not produce large amounts of adrenalin on a normal basis. That's why exercise will help those people to increase their adrenalin production and thus exercise the heart. It's also why you will look around at the people who are in your life and wonder why they don't have the problems you do while drinking and eating the foul stuff that they do."

"Actually, I was going to ask you about that. Other people eat sweets, do caffeine and artificial sweeteners, and live a high stress life as I do, but they don't have the problems that I have."

"That's because they are not born as high adrenalin producers in the first place. Lyn, there are some people that are born making large amounts of adrenalin as their normal production. It's a genetic thing. You have no control over that, and neither do I. Nothing will change your genetic make-up. The majority of people are not born 'movers and shakers.' That's what I have always called high-adrenalin producers. The majority of people make significantly less amounts of adrenalin than you do in the very same situation.

"Therefore, they will not exhibit the signs of adrenal fatigue as quickly as you will. They certainly can and do end up where you are when their adrenal stimulant intake grows to such a level that the adrenals are worn to a frazzle, but it will take them longer to get there than for you under the same circumstances."

"That doesn't seem fair," Lyn commented.

"Actually, I see the genetically high-adrenalin producers as blessed. Those additional amounts of everyday adrenalin give these people a very sharp and quick mind. They are able to understand concepts rapidly and thoroughly.

They have the potential to be geniuses."

"But they eventually get all the trouble of adrenal fatigue," Lyn said.

"That's only if they don't take care of themselves. If the genetically high-adrenalin producers did the lists that I am going to give you today, they would never reach adrenal fatigue. They would live their lives out to the full without aches and pains, depression, anxiety, arthritis, and fibromyalgia, as well as a host of other disorders that come with adrenal fatigue. They would live life more completely."

"That's what I want. Vibrancy in life—and no pain. No rheumatoid arthritis. No ulcerative colitis."

"That's where we're going, Lyn," Karen said. "That's where we're going."

CHAPTER 10

Adrenal Helpers

"Are we ready for 'the lists' yet?" Lyn asked.

"Not quite. I have spent a lot of time educating you on the things that stress the adrenal glands, but now I need to tell you the things that will help us build the adrenals. It's one thing to take away the whips that we have used to beat those glands into a pulp, but we need something to aid us in recovering these bludgeoned horses.

"The first is something that you'll already be doing for your ulcerative colitis. That is soluble fiber. Remember how the soluble fiber will remove bile from the gastrointestinal tract?"

"Yes, and then the liver will make new bile," Lyn answered.

"Correct. And the new bile is less saturated with waste products each time we have run a batch through the system," Karen said. "But here's the connection with the need of soluble fiber and rheumatoid arthritis—the adrenal hormones are cleared by the liver and deposited into the bile."

"I thought the bile was the liver's dumping ground for garbage," Lyn said.

"It is, however, adrenal hormones as well as all other hormones are filtered out of the blood by the liver. The liver has to get rid of these hormones just as much as it has to rid the body of circulating toxins. So the hormones are deposited in the bile."

"You mean I have adrenalin-laced bile?"

"You do."

"But I thought I wasn't making *enough* adrenalin and corticosteroids," Lyn protested.

"For a good majority of the time, you aren't. But you are not adrenalin-less or totally corticosteroid-less. You still make these hormones, but not in sufficient amounts on a consistent basis. You're like a light switch. When you take in an adrenal stimulant such as sugar or caffeine, the adrenals are forced to produce large amounts of hormones. This is like the light switch being fully on. The liver will clear these large amounts of hormones, dumping them into the bile. Then you don't have sufficient amounts of the hormones in the bloodstream. That's like the light switch being off. Either you're on or off—with nothing much in between."

"That's exactly how I feel. I'm either functioning in a short blaze of glory or I'm groveling in the dark."

"Yep. But that's about to change. It'll take a bit longer to heal from the rheumatoid arthritis than from the ulcerative colitis, but we'll be able to get those adrenals humming along at optimum and without the use of whips." Karen paused, "That is *if* you cooperate."

"Can't you tell that I'm chomping at the bit to get to those lists? I'm ready to do anything to rid myself of the daily misery that I'm in."

Karen laughed. "I can tell. But if I don't tell you the 'why' of items that will be included in your lists, you will be less likely to stick to them."

"Okay. Tell me why I need beans to help my rheumatoid arthritis."

"The beans carry out the hormones being cleared by the liver. We need to help the endocrine system by not recycling old hormones that are in the bile.

"I want to go back to this issue of the production of hormones. You need to understand that you still *do* make hormones. They are just not the right amount at the right time. You're like an old-time jalopy that's going down the road. You're moving forward at all times, but the engine sputters and backfires. You jerk along more than glide along. It's not a smooth ride. Sputter, sputter, clunk, clunk, jerk, jolt, shudder, twitch—the old jalopy moves along—but it doesn't move along well."

"I get it."

"When we recycle the hormone-laden bile we just add more inconsistency to the delicate and precise balance of hormone levels that the pituitary is trying to achieve."

"Aren't these hormones in the bile caught and imprisoned there?" Lyn asked.

"No. It would be helpful if they were encapsulated in the bile in such a way that they could not cause any bodily response. But they aren't. When bile is absorbed through the small intestine, it is the components of the bile that we find retracing the bloodstream: the fatty acids, the toxins, the hormones—they are all back to a free float wreaking havoc in the bloodstream. The liver filters the bile back out of the bloodstream by the bile's constituent parts. For simplicity's sake, I usually just say the bile returns to the liver, allowing the assumption that the very bile is flowing through the blood vessels and arrives at its destination of the liver. But in actuality—it is the little bitty parts that make up the bile that are retracing the bloodstream."

"So that's another reason why it's so important to toss the bile into the toilet," Lyn concluded.

"Yes, because if we don't toss the bile constituents away, they run wild and free again in our bloodstream until the liver can catch them. This fouls the delicate negative-feedback system of the pituitary which is constantly doing a complicated dance with all the endocrine glands as well as the hypothalamus. It's an incredibly complex system and the return of the nasties as well as the return of the hormones from the trash heap causes glitches in the system."

Lyn said, "I like your illustration about the old car. I do feel like I'm hiccupping down the road, lurching forward and then dropping back, only to hiccup again."

"Your jalopy jerk has got to stop," Karen responded, "so we'll use soluble fiber to help us in this process. If we keep the trash and old hormones from returning to the bloodstream then the higher authorities—which are the hypothalamus and pituitary—can keep the balance without dealing with renegades."

"I got it," Lyn said.

"Good. Then I'll move on to the next critical factor in recovering those adrenals. Protein."

Lyn interjected, "Oh, I get plenty of that. Peanut butter and cheese are some of my favorite foods."

Karen smiled. Lyn's statement was typical. Almost everyone thought that peanut butter and cheese were good sources of protein. "I hate to burst your bubble, but those two foods will not help us very much. They are not bad foods, but they will not be able to accomplish the work that we need to do. They are not efficient proteins."

"Karen, I'm certain that peanut butter and cheese have protein."

"They are a source of protein, but we need to classify what a 'good' source of protein is."

"You told me that I wouldn't have to eat lizard tails and fish eyes!"

"You won't. It'll be regular food, and peanut butter and cheese will certainly be allowed—after a time, since we have ulcerative colitis that must be dealt with also—but peanut butter and cheese will not heal your endocrine system. And *that* must be done to cure your rheumatoid arthritis.

"Let me explain proteins. First, know that a protein is made up of amino acids. I'll use the English alphabet as an example to help you see clearly. To make a word we need letters. We have twenty-six letters in the alphabet. If we remove all the vowels: a, e, i, o, u, and the occasionally used vowels w and y, how many words can we make?"

Lyn did not even hesitate. The answer was obvious. "None."

"It is similar with protein. To make a protein molecule we need letters which are in reality amino acids. There are certain amino acids that are *essential*. Please note I said essential, not efficient. These essential amino acids are like the vowels. If we remove them from the amino acid alphabet, we cannot make any proteins. The consonants in the amino acid alphabet are called non-essential. If we have a food that has all of the essential amino acids present, then we say that we have a *complete* protein.

"But a complete protein is only one criterion in evaluating the worth of protein foods. A second criterion is whether a complete protein is efficient or inefficient."

"Hold on. So eating beans and rice together is not good?" Lyn asked. "I've heard that if a person combines different foods they make it a good protein."

"Eating beans and rice is not bad. However, food combining may make a *complete* protein, but not necessarily a 'good' or more specifically an *efficient* protein," Karen responded. "Hang with me now so that I can make this clear."

"Okay, I'll be quiet and listen."

"Let's pretend that you are very hungry, Lyn. Let's also pretend that I am responsible for providing your food. You really want a turkey sandwich. I say, 'No problem,' and I leave and return shortly with a turkey sandwich which I place in front of you. You eat it ravenously. It hits the spot. Your appetite is satisfied.

"Then the next day you tell me again, 'I'd like a turkey sandwich.' I say 'No problem.' But this time I disappear and return with a bag of wheat berries. I plop them down in front of you while pointing out the window. 'You see that turkey that's running loose in the yard?' You look at me with big round eyes, but I ignore you. 'Here are the wheat berries. There's the turkey. You see, I have provided for you. You make the effort to put together your turkey sandwich.'"

"Okay, I'm beginning to understand."

Karen drove the point home. "The already-made turkey sandwich is like the efficient protein—one that the body utilizes well and immediately. The inefficient protein—even if it is complete—is the bag of wheat berries and the live turkey. Certainly all the building blocks are there, but we put the body through hoops to arrive at the end product. It's so much simpler to just eat the efficient protein. Not only simpler, but efficient proteins will build our health rapidly."

Lyn objected, "But I always thought eating lots of protein wasn't that good for a person."

"All human tissue, all cells, are made from protein. Without protein, we would cease to exist," Karen said. "It is this very protein, *efficient* protein, that will aid us in rebuilding your adrenals. Your adrenal cells are protein.

"As far as eating too much protein—that's pretty hard to do unless you limited your diet to nothing but protein with no carbohydrates. Then we move into the ketosis state that I explained to you earlier. But this is an extreme and not the norm. Believe me, I will never ask you to eat so much protein that you will strain your liver and kidneys with ketosis. But you will eat much more protein than you are currently consuming."

"What are the efficient proteins?" Lyn asked.

"There are only five. They are: eggs, meat, poultry, fish, and seafood."

Lyn was still resistant. "But what about the fat in these foods? That can't be good for you."

"Fats are just as necessary as proteins for sustaining life. In fact, the hormones that those adrenal cells make are made out of fats. But you are right in this: some fats are not as good for you as others.

"I'll be asking you to eat meat and poultry that is lean. So we will have as little bad fat as possible. Fish and seafood have very good fats that we desperately need; and eggs are not at all bad as far as fats go."

Lyn balked. "It's known everywhere that eggs are bad for a person because of the cholesterol."

"That's what has been assumed and unfortunately taught throughout many years; however, there is now evidence to show that the cholesterol found in the yolk of an egg does not affect blood cholesterol levels."

"I don't get it. If there's cholesterol in an egg yolk and we eat the egg, the cholesterol should land in the blood," Lyn said.

"Actually, that is a reasonable line of logic. In fact, it was this thinking that put eggs on the 'bad' list in the beginning. When it was discovered that increased levels of bad cholesterol in the bloodstream contributed to heart disease, the assumption was made that any food that contained cholesterol would automatically add to this problem. Based on this rational train of thought, recommendations were made to the public to cease or at least decrease the consumption of eggs.

"But the testing of this hypothesis—that eggs contribute to increased cholesterol levels—was not complete at that time. It takes years to gather data and conduct studies. Now several decades later, the test results are coming in. The conclusions are that eggs do *not* necessarily affect blood cholesterol levels. In fact, in some studies, people who did not eat eggs had higher blood cholesterol levels than those who ate eggs every day.[6]"

It was hard for Lyn to accept this. "But I even remember seeing a poster in the doctor's office that talked about not eating eggs."

Karen replied patiently. "We are only humankind. And humankind, as hard as it tries, is prone to mistakes. It was a reasonable mistake to make. It does seem logical to assume that eating foods that have cholesterol in them will raise blood cholesterol; however, there are many bodily functions that come into play in metabolizing fats. It is complicated and we are just now learning more about this.

"It's extremely interesting to me the role that sugars play in the fat levels in the bloodstream. Sugars are converted into fats that actually account for a significant portion of our total cholesterol level. They are known as triglycerides."

---

[6] See appendix for further remarks and references.

Karen continued. "If it brings you any comfort, the legumes that you will be eating will prevent absorption of fats from the intestinal tract, including cholesterol. So if the conclusions of the studies are wrong, and eggs are found to absolutely raise blood cholesterol, the consumption of beans along with your eggs will prevent the cholesterol found in that yolk from entering your bloodstream."

"But I thought the legumes were supposed to bind with bile," Lyn said.

"They do. But the soluble fiber in the legumes also binds with the fats that we consume at that same meal. Beans are fat sponges. They soak up the fats—whether good or bad—and toss them into the toilet."

"I never knew that beans were so good for people."

"Most people don't."

"I have a feeling that beans are going to appear on my list several times," Lyn ventured.

"They will."

"But Karen, beans cause gas, and I can't afford to spread that type of perfume around my work place."

"Beans don't cause gas. They take gas away," Karen replied.

"But what about the little rhyme: 'Beans, beans, the magical fruit, the more you eat the more you toot,'" Lyn said.

"You didn't finish the rhyme," Karen laughed. "'The more you toot, the better you feel, so eat some beans at every meal!'"

Lyn laughed too. "Okay. So now tell me how beans are not responsible for tooting."

"It might help if I tell you a true story about one of my clients. A young man from Canada contacted me because of the tremendous gas problems that he had. He had been suffering with extreme flatulence for several years. It was to the point that he was in such pain that he would at times be doubled over in agony and couldn't even go to work.

"I spent quite some time explaining to him the workings of the gastrointestinal tract and the role of bile, the recycling of bile, and the results of that recycling before coming to the conclusion: 'you'll have to eat beans to cure yourself of the flatulence.'

"The man immediately responded with vehemence, 'I will *not* eat a bean. They *cause* gas. I haven't eaten beans in years!' I quietly responded, 'If beans cause gas, and you have not eaten a bean in years, then what in the world is causing your gas?'

"That took the wind out of his sails and after he sputtered and muttered for a bit, I explained the 'why.' It is bile that causes gas. Nasty, recycled bile ferments our foods instead of digesting them. Fermentation always has a by-product of gas. If the bile was mild—not saturated with trash that has been recycling for who-knows-how-long—then we will have digestion take place, not fermentation. The only way to keep bile from recycling is to consume soluble fiber."

"But it really seems that beans do cause gas. Whenever people eat them, they do start to toot," Lyn insisted.

"Remember how I told you that bile is very attracted to soluble fiber?" Karen asked.

"Yes."

"When beans enter the duodenum, bile will immediately unbind with whatever it is currently bound. It will rush to the soluble fiber and form a permanent bond with it. Foul bile ferments everything, including beans! Bile is going to ferment something—whatever it binds with—no matter what type of bond, permanent or temporary. If beans attract the bile over any other food, then the beans will be a target for fermentation. We will have gas until the bile is made mild.

"The less nasty the bile is, the less fermentation takes place, therefore the less gas is produced. So if we can get the bile to be less noxious, then we won't have fermentation. The only way to accomplish this is to force the exit of the bile into the toilet so that the liver has a chance to make brand-new mild bile. So a person . . ."

"Has to eat their beans," Lyn finished. "But Karen, I can't believe that soluble fiber is the only thing that causes bile to leave the body. There has to be something else."

Karen laughed loudly. "There is!"

"What's so funny?!" Lyn demanded.

"It's you! That's how we dump bile if there are no beans!"

"I don't get it," Lyn said sourly. "And I'm not laughing."

"I'm sorry," Karen said as she tried to stifle her mirth. "When I said, 'It's you,' I meant it's your very problem with diarrhea. If we have nasty bile that has to be dumped and there is no soluble fiber to facilitate this action, there is only one course of action left: don't give the bile time to absorb at the ileum which translates to—diarrhea."

Lyn sighed. If she had only known all this information before! Maybe she could have been saved a lot of her misery.

Karen was still speaking. "Yes, yes. Beans. Lots of beans. But now, Lyn, there is more that I have to teach you about rebuilding your adrenals so that we can conquer rheumatoid arthritis. I was talking to you about the need for efficient proteins, including eggs with their much maligned cholesterol. You'll be able to eat the efficient proteins without worrying about the cholesterol because you'll be eating beans alongside them."

Lyn interrupted, "Wait, before you go on I want to know what happened to the man from Canada? Did he eat the beans?"

"He did. I had told him to call me in two weeks. By then he should be seeing results and I would want to talk with him to establish a maintenance plan. But in one week I received a call from him. He said he couldn't wait another week to tell me. He had begun the legumes immediately after we first talked. Within three days he had no gas for the first time in years. The pain was gone and he felt like a new person."

"Wow. That was fast. Only three days," Lyn remarked.

Karen agreed. "Three days is a quick heal, but he was in his early twenties. I have found that the younger a person is the faster the results. For an older person, it usually takes a while longer—but it still works."

"Maybe I'll heal quickly. I'm barely thirty."

"You probably will as long as you stick to the lists. If you deviate from the lists, then your healing will be slower and not as effective. I'll remind you when we get there. But I'll say it now also: no cheats, Lyn, no cheats!"

"I'll be a good girl, I promise!"

Karen smiled. "Back to summarizing proteins: to get the adrenals to function at optimum, you will have to consume adequate amounts of the efficient proteins. I'll be specific about amounts when we get to the lists.

"Next thing: there is an element in healing the adrenals that is just as critical as your diet. This one deals with your lifestyle. It is rest."

"That's not a problem. I average six to seven hours a night."

"Well, you're right up there with the average American, but that is an insufficient amount of sleep. It's not enough for regular good health, and a far cry from what we'll need to cure your problems. For most healthy people eight hours of sleep is necessary. But how much sleep a person needs depends on two major factors: how high an adrenalin-producer they are and if they are currently ill. The more adrenalin that a person makes on an everyday basis, the more sleep is necessary, and if a person is fighting any kind of illness—including rheumatoid arthritis or ulcerative colitis, more sleep is necessary to facilitate the healing process."

Lyn was tapping her pen on her pad. "Interesting. I had never thought about that before."

"Actually, for your rheumatoid arthritis, sleep will be the critical factor. If you do the eating plan exactly as I spell out, but do not get your sleep, you will never completely heal from the arthritis. Remember that rheumatoid arthritis, in my theory, is caused by a lack of corticosteroid production. That deficit in these anti-inflammatory hormones is caused by a fatigued adrenal system. When a gland is fatigued, rest is absolutely essential to recover it."

"It makes sense. But sometimes I'm not able to sleep, or I toss and turn, or I have wild and weird dreams. I often wake up feeling just as tired as when I went to bed."

Karen replied, "Not sleeping well is usually a function of too much adrenalin at the wrong time. It can also be the pain that keeps you awake. Either way, both of these problems will resolve as you begin to eat differently. We'll be removing the adrenal whips which eventually will solve the busy brain syndrome and the toss-and-turn behavior."

"Busy brain syndrome?" Lyn asked.

"That's what I call it when a person lies awake at night with their brain thinking at a hundred miles an hour. They're thinking so much about all kinds of things that they can't sleep."

"How does removing the adrenal whips stop that?"

"Remember that adrenalin is made of two incredibly powerful neurotransmitters—epinephrine and norepinephrine. These neurotransmitters allow more messages to cross the neural synapses than any other neurotransmitter, causing you to think more and think faster. Busy brain," Karen concluded.

"So if I don't stimulate adrenal production then I won't lie awake as much."

Karen answered, "That's it. And you won't toss and turn so much. Being a light sleeper is another indication of too much adrenalin at the wrong time. If the neural gaps are filled with this potent neurotransmitter while you are asleep, then you are 'thinking' while sleeping which makes for the restlessness. It also creates crazy dreams."

Lyn wanted to know right away and couldn't keep from asking, "How much sleep are you going to recommend?"

"For you, based on your current status of health—or I should say 'ill-health'—ten hours for every twenty-four that pass."

"Karen, I don't know that I'll be able to do that. I can't sleep that long," Lyn protested. She added in a small voice, "Although I'd like to try. I always seem so very tired."

"If you cannot sleep it, I'll need you to 'rest' it."

"Does reading or watching TV count as resting?" Lyn inquired.

"No. The only resting that counts is quietly reclining with your eyes closed—whether you are sleeping or not," Karen answered.

"Wow. This means I'm going to have to revamp my whole schedule."

"This sleep/rest requirement is usually the hardest thing for people to conquer. But it will have to be done if you are to see a cure to your rheumatoid arthritis."

"I get goose bumps every time you say that."

"Say what?" Karen asked.

"That there's a cure for rheumatoid arthritis. It's so hard for me to believe. They've always said that it wasn't possible."

Karen didn't answer right away. How many times had she heard this before from hundreds and hundreds of clients? How many times had she herself been told that it wasn't possible?

Karen quietly responded, "If Columbus had believed the current teachings of his day, it wouldn't have been possible for him to prove that the world was round. If the Wright brothers had listened to the scholarly advice of the day, they would have never flown that first plane at Kitty Hawk. If believing something was impossible dictated its reality, then we never would have seen a man walking on the moon. I am no different in my studies than Columbus or the Wright brothers. *They* may say that it's not possible, but I don't ascribe to that line of reasoning."

Karen did not give Lyn a chance to respond to this speech but fixed the final tack in the posting of the notice about the need for rest. "Lyn, there's another thing that you have to do to rest your adrenal glands besides getting ten hours of sleep/rest. You must allow yourself to take off one day of work each week."

"Oh, I already do that," Lyn responded blithely. "I don't have to work Saturday or Sunday."

"I didn't phrase it very well," Karen responded. "I mean that I need you to rest one day out of seven."

"You mean I have to sleep for one entire day each week?" Lyn was taken aback.

"No, I mean that you aren't supposed to go to work at your job, or go to work at your home, or go to work anywhere. Your adrenal glands need one day a week that they don't have to rise to the occasion by producing large amounts of adrenalin to get you through whatever activity you're doing."

"What does resting mean? How is this different from the ten hours of sleep/rest?"

"Resting one day out of the week means reading a book, watching a movie, sitting on the back porch idly observing the hummingbirds at the feeder. It means low activity. This day of rest will not be the day to mop the kitchen floor, catch up on the laundry, pay the bills, and otherwise do the things that you didn't get done during the work-week."

"Does it matter which day of the week?" Lyn asked.

"No. Just one day out of every seven Lyn Redmond needs to be lounging about."

"Will I ever be able to cut back on the amount of rest?"

"In time, your sleep requirement of ten hours will be reduced, but for your optimal health the taking-it-easy day should always be kept in place."

Lyn sighed. "Okay, if the adrenals need to rest to heal, I'll rest them."

Karen summarized, "Now you know the importance of legumes, efficient proteins, and rest in the building of the endocrine system—specifically in your case, the building of the adrenals. Now we are ready for 'the lists.'"

11

CHAPTER 11

The Lists

"Yes! We're finally to the lists," Lyn said with anticipation. "I've been waiting to hear this. When you first talked about them, I was afraid of the tortuous 'lists', but now I just want to know exactly what I have to do to get out of this dark hole that I'm in."

Karen answered, "I'm not sorry for the time that I had to take to explain everything to you. If I started with the lists, you would have probably rejected them outright. Without knowledge, there is only suspicion."

"I understand and agree," Lyn said. "Now, Karen, don't put me off any longer. What are the lists?"

"We'll start with the 'No' list. Everything on this list is targeted to stop stressing your endocrine system and to stop aggravating your rheumatoid arthritis and ulcerative colitis.

The "No" List

1. Sweets—this means no desserts such as cakes, pies, cookies, candy, doughnuts, muffins, sweet breads (i.e. zucchini bread, pumpkin bread, banana bread), jello, pudding, ice cream, granola bars or anything that you know is a sweet.

2. Natural sweeteners—this means no jam, jelly, honey, syrup (even if it is 100% pure maple syrup), molasses, brown sugar, raw sugar, or natural sweetener of any kind.

3. Artificial sweeteners—this means no aspartame which is also known as Nutrasweet, saccharin, Sweet N Low, Equal, Splenda, Stevia, sugar alcohols (i.e. mannitol, sorbitol, xylitol, maltitol), or any artificial or so-called 'natural-artificial' sweetener.

4. Caffeine—this means no coffee, caffeinated teas, chocolate, or soda.

5. Decaffeinated products.

6. Sweetened beverages of any kind—this means no soda *of any kind*, lemonade, punches, hot chocolate, ciders, or any other beverage that is sweet.

7. Fruit juice—this means all fruit juice—even 100% natural fruit juice.

8. Fruit—until you are well—then we will allow you one piece of fruit daily.

9. Fragrances or perfumes of any kind—this includes hand soaps, dish soaps, shampoos, hair conditioners, body lotions, laundry soap, air fresheners, scented candles, potpourri, aroma therapy, or other scented products.

10. No formal exercise.

Karen paused to summarize this part of the list. "All the above items are specifically included as they are the major offenders to the endocrine system."

"These are the whips?" Lyn asked.

"Yes, these are the substances that have worn your system down to the point that you are unable to make adequate adrenalin for 'zippety-do-dah' and neither are you able to make the corticosteroids to prevent the inflammation that occurs daily from friction—thus your arthritis."

"Okay. Go on."

"Before I continue the 'No' list I need to warn you about something. Because everything on the list that I have compiled for you so far is an adrenal whip—you must be prepared for withdrawal."

"Withdrawal? From sugar and fruit?"

"And caffeine, artificial sweeteners, fragrances, and exercise," Karen responded. "Remember that years ago you fatigued the adrenals to the point that you *needed* the whips to make them function at a normal level. So for a long time you have relied on the very substances that created this fatigue to force your glands to work harder. And even now, you are reliant on these whips for what inadequate function that you do have.

"We are pulling out all the whips. Nothing is going to drive your horses to greater achievement. The horses that are pulling your wagon will stand stock-still. You won't die or anything like that, but you won't have the adrenalin or corticosteroid production that you now have, as insufficient as that amount is."

Lyn almost moaned. "You're telling me that I'm going to feel worse—not better."

"I am. But it's only for two weeks. Withdrawal normally doesn't take much longer than that."

"What should I expect?" Lyn asked.

"Headaches, more joint aches than you currently experience, extreme fatigue, irritability, and even heart palpitations. But none of it is dangerous, just inconvenient."

"Sounds like I should lock myself in a closet for two weeks."

Karen laughed. "It won't be *that* bad, but you won't exactly be feeling chipper."

"Alright," Lyn sighed, "I'm forewarned."

"Then on to the remainder of the 'No' list," Karen said. "These items are very specific for you at this moment in time because you are experiencing the rage of bloody ulcerative colitis. This part of the 'No' list will change rapidly as you heal over the next several days. In fact, I'll want to talk to you in exactly one week. By then, some things will have already changed."

"Good. It seems like I'm spending my life in the bathroom. I'd like to see that changed right away," Lyn said.

"Ulcerative colitis we can change immediately. Healing the endocrine system will take us longer—but the bowels will respond rapidly. Here's the rest of your 'No' list."

Lyn's "No" List Continued

11. Dairy—this means no milk, cheese, butter, yogurt, sour cream, or dairy product of any kind.
12. Cruciferous vegetables—this means no broccoli, cauliflower, cabbage, Brussels sprouts, rutabaga, turnips or radishes—cooked or uncooked.
13. Raw vegetables of any kind.
14. Corn of any kind.
15. Acidic foods—this means no tomato sauce, pizza sauce, salsas, vinegar, or hot spices.
16. Nuts.
17. Seeds.
18. Nut or seed butters—this means no peanut butter, almond butter, cashew butter, sesame seed butter, etc.
19. Condiments—this means no mayonnaise, mustard, ketchup, salad dressings, etc.
20. Whole grain products.
21. Teas of any kind, even if they are caffeine-free.
22. Multi-vitamin or supplements of any kind.
23. Hunger.

"Stop, stop," Lyn interrupted. "You have to explain why no multi-vitamins or supplements are allowed."

"Multi-vitamins, overall, are good things, but not for you at this time. The B vitamins in the multi will only stimulate a bile release which will cause more gut irritation. In time, we'll add the multi-vitamin back," Karen answered. "As far as supplements go, it would depend upon the exact supplement, but most of them will have one or more ingredients that could aggravate the ulcerative colitis. Even certain types of calcium products will aggravate the gut, even though pure calcium is known to sooth the gastro-intestinal tract. It's the other ingredients that come with the calcium that will be offensive. We simply can't risk any irritants right now."

"And what did you mean by 'hunger'?" Lyn asked.

"You are not allowed to be hungry. If you become hungry, it means that we permitted your blood glucose levels to fall which in turn will kick in an adrenal response to facilitate the release of liver glycogen. We can't tolerate that right now. We have too much healing to do. Being hungry will slow us down."

"So, I get to eat all that I want?" Lyn asked.

"Yes," Karen replied, "of the things on your 'Do' list which I am ready to give you, if you're ready."

"Wait, two more questions. Why no whole grains?"

"Because of the high insoluble fiber content. This type of fiber is like a little scrub brush on your tender open sores in the gastro-intestinal tract. We don't want that right now. In time, I'll be telling you to eat whole grain products—but not today. Maybe in a few weeks. We'll see how quickly you heal."

"And why no caffeine-free teas?"

"Teas have tannins that usually do not irritate, however, if the gastro-intestinal tract is already severely aggravated as yours is, oftentimes the tannic acids will exacerbate the situation."

Lyn was writing as fast as she could. After a pause Karen said, "Ready for the 'Do' list now?"

"Yes," replied Lyn.

"This list will change fairly rapidly, maybe even in the next few weeks, depending on whether you are still experiencing the bloody stools. I'll adjust this list, as well as the 'No' list based on your progress."

The "Do" List

1. You must eat one-half cup of legumes six times daily. This means you will eat one-half cup beans for breakfast, for a mid-morning snack, for lunch, for a mid-afternoon snack, for dinner, and for a bedtime snack. Do not try to combine the servings and decrease the frequency. It is the frequency that is priority, not the serving size. In other words, don't eat one cup of beans for breakfast thinking that you will take care of the mid-morning snack of beans at the same time. It doesn't work that way. Bile continually drips into your duodenum. I want to bind and carry out bile six different times in a day—not five or four or three. Six! Now if you want to eat more than the one-half of a cup of beans for breakfast, you may. The one-half cup is only a minimum. You may eat all the beans you want at one sitting, but you will have to eat them again at mid-morning and the rest of the times in the day to reach the total of having consumed beans six different times each day.

   Legumes are beans such as pinto, kidney, garbanzo, Great Northern, navy, lentils, limas, black beans, brown beans, white beans, red beans, black-eyed peas, yellow-eyes peas, pigeon peas, green split peas, and yellow split peas. There are more types of legumes also but too many to list. Just remember for our purposes, green beans, wax beans, soy beans, and peanuts do not qualify as legumes.

2. You must eat a minimum of three to four ounces of efficient protein at breakfast, at lunch, and again at dinner. The efficient proteins are eggs, meat, poultry, fish, and seafood. Lyn, your efficient proteins must be lean. No fatty foods for you right now. Three to four ounces is roughly equivalent to the size of a deck of cards.

3. You must drink one-half gallon of either distilled or reverse osmosis water each day. One-half gallon is sixty-four fluid ounces or eight cups. We cannot afford to drink water that is not purified as the chlorine in tap

water, as well as other contaminants, can be aggravating to your gastrointestinal system.

4. You absolutely must sleep/rest for ten hours a day. It does not have to be consecutive. You may sleep nine hours at night and take a one hour nap in the day or any combination of naps and rests, so long as you reach the ten hours in that day.

5. You must rest one day out of every seven. You don't have to sleep the whole day, but you must rest.

"Now we're ready for the 'Allowed' list," Karen said.

"Isn't there more on the 'Do' list?" Lyn asked. "It's not very long."

"It will get a little longer once we pass the first stage of healing. But the purpose of the 'Do' list is to make sure you eat those things that will facilitate your recovery. Those things must be accomplished without fail. The allowed list will contain things that you may eat. They are neither harmful nor necessarily helpful, but certainly can be eaten."

"So I *have* to eat the things on the 'Do' list, and I *may* eat the things on the 'Allowed' list," Lyn said.

"You got it," Karen answered. "Here's your 'Allowed' list for today. Keep in mind that this list will also change as we progress.

The "Allowed" List

1. Well-cooked vegetables that are not crucifers.

2. White bread, white crackers, white noodles, white potatoes (no skins), white rice, 'white' cereals such as crisped rice, puffed rice, crisped wheat, puffed wheat, cream of rice cereal or cream of wheat cereal. These foods comprise what I have termed the 'White Diet.' They require little digestive work allowing your intestinal tract to rest and giving the sores on the intestinal wall a chance to heal.

3. Broths, as long as they are not highly seasoned.

"You can see, Lyn, that I have pulled almost all the fibers and fats out of your diet. This is necessary to allow your open ulcers to heal. Fibers are essential to the health of the intestinal tract, but not as this time. Fats are also essential to hormone production, but until we clear up the gut problem, the fats will only create more havoc there."

"I understand," Lyn replied.

Karen said, "This completes the lists. Now it's time to begin. Remember, no cheating. Follow the rules."

"What about my medications?" Lyn asked.

"Stay on them until we see progress. I'll recommend weaning off of them at the appropriate time, and you can then check with your doctor to see if he agrees."

"It'll be great if I can get rid of those enemas and suppositories," Lyn said.

"That's on my list of goals, too," Karen responded. "Now, Lyn, I want to talk to you in one week. We should already be seeing some changes by then. Let's set up a time."

As Lyn hung up the phone, she felt hope like she had not felt in a long time. She immediately began making up a grocery list.

12

CHAPTER 12

The Road to Recovery

It was a beautiful summer day when exactly one week later Lyn was on the phone at the appointed time for her follow-up. The warm but not overly hot weather, as well as the brilliantly green landscape that made Wisconsin famous for its summers, added to the sense of optimism that pervaded Lyn's attitude.

"I had a total of three headaches this past week," Lyn reported.

"But you stayed clean and didn't succumb to drinking your soda, right?" Karen asked.

"I am squeaky clean," Lyn answered. "Absolutely no cheats. I did everything on the lists with the exception of the ten hours of sleep. I'm certainly better on the sleep than I ever was in the past, but I'm not quite there yet."

"Keep working on that angle. That's one of the critical pieces for curing the rheumatoid arthritis. Sorry about the headaches, but that's all part of withdrawal. Remember it takes two weeks."

Lyn replied, "I haven't forgotten. I'm staying the course despite the rascally headaches."

"Good. Now tell me about the bowels," Karen said.

"I'm down to four to five bowel movements a day instead of the eight or nine. The stools are more formed and less little pieces, and the abdominal cramping is less. And I'm not having any of those stools that are just pure blood."

"But you still have some blood in the stools?" Karen asked.

"Yes, but not as much."

Karen nodded although Lyn couldn't see that across the phone lines. "You're coming along nicely. Now, have you lost weight? I expect about a three to five pound weight loss this past week."

"Yes, I lost three pounds. I was wondering if that was normal," Lyn said.

"Absolutely normal. As we're able to add more things to your 'Do' and 'Allowed' list, you'll stop losing, but for now be prepared that you may lose a little bit more. Though it won't be but a few pounds more."

"That's fine with me. I'd like to lose a couple more pounds."

Karen replied, "I will draw a line though. Being too thin is just as bad as being too thick. But you're 129 pounds on a small five foot six inch frame, so you're okay. I'd even let you go down to 120 pounds, but no lower than that."

Karen talked to Lyn for several more minutes, answering her questions about green peppers—"absolutely not"—and asparagus tips—"certainly"—before instructing Lyn to continue the original lists. She set up another time to talk to Lyn in two weeks.

* * * * * * *

"It's August twenty-fourth, so three weeks now. I'm not seeing the progress that I want to see. So, Lyn, I'm going to pull all the vegetables out," Karen said as Lyn finished her report.

Although her stools were more formed and the frequency was reduced from the original eight or nine bloody stools to an average of six, it was still not where they needed to be. Too many "gas and spatter" bowel movements as Lyn called them, and still too much blood. Lyn was being faithful to the diet and also taking her medications religiously, but it was time to be even stricter.

"It was the wild rice that gave me the 'gas and spatters,'" Lyn was saying. "But I'm only having the intestinal cramping right before a bowel movement, not any other time."

"Are you able to hold the enema or are you expelling it immediately?" Karen asked.

"Expelling it immediately," Lyn answered.

"Okay. We run an even tighter ship now," Karen replied. "Absolutely no fat and absolutely no insoluble fiber. You eat the White Diet with the addition of eggs and the white meat of chicken. No fish, no protein that has fat. Your life is just legumes, white starches, eggs, chicken, and water. And I want to talk to you in one week."

Lyn was willing to do whatever Karen recommended. She was really quite pleased that she had fewer blow-outs each day. It was more progress than she had ever seen before, so she was willing to cut back to the things that Karen was recommending.

* * * * * * *

The week passed. Lyn could hardly believe the things herself as she reported them to Karen. It was September second.

"I have had no blood in my stool since August twenty-seventh, three days after we last talked," Lyn said. "And I have had no intestinal cramping since August twenty-sixth! My bowel movements are large and formed, and I am able to retain the enema!"

"Excellent. You're where you are supposed to be now," Karen replied. "Let's add back the well-cooked vegetables. No more than one serving per meal though. And Lyn, it's time for you to call your physician and inquire about dropping the enema treatment."

* * * * * * *

Another week passed before Karen spoke with Lyn again.

Lyn said, "I'm down to two bowel movements a day. Still no blood, still no diarrhea, still no cramping. The doctor said I could drop the enema but would need to take the suppositories both in the morning and the evening. He also told me that it would be impossible for me to ever come off the suppositories. He's glad that I have progressed this far, but doesn't believe I'll truly be able to cure my ulcerative colitis."

"We have nothing to prove to anyone, Lyn. We simply need to continue working to get you 100% well. Whether your doctor believes it can happen or not won't affect what we're doing. We press or."

"Karen, I haven't had to take any Vioxx for weeks. I get pain here and there but I don't take anything for it. I just deal with it. It is *nothing* like it used to be."

"This is a bonus, Lyn. Normally it takes longer for us to see improvement with the arthritis. You're progressing rapidly. Outstanding!"

* * * * * * *

In two weeks Lyn called to check in again.

"Lyn, your report is excellent. Not only have you had no rheumatoid arthritis flare-ups, but you have no symptoms of ulcerative colitis. We have added back in all the foods now, including the cooked cruciferous, cheese, and nut butters. We only have the raw vegetables and fruit to add back into your diet. When we can successfully add these back in, then we will look at withdrawal from those suppositories."

"I'm nervous about the raw vegetables. It's been so wonderful to not worry about running to the bathroom. Karen, I have no cramping, no blood—nothing—just normal bowel movements. I don't want to lose that."

"I understand. Let's wait a week before we test the waters with the raw vegetables."

* * * * * * *

Lyn's week was going so well that she decided to drop the morning suppository. She knew that Karen would be supportive as long as she had tried those raw vegetables and had no problems. So first, she spent a few days with raw vegetables added to her diet, and had no negative effects. Hurray! Now, no more morning suppository. She went through the days with bated breath, waiting to see if she would have to do the run-to-the-bathroom exercise, but she never did. When her appointment time with Karen came, she was ecstatic.

"Karen, no morning suppository for a week now and I've had no problems. The raw vegetables are going down well, though I'm not eating any tomatoes yet. And I am feeling so wonderful! I have so much energy!"

Karen could imagine Lyn twirling about the room. "I really do have a cool job," she thought to herself. It was so rewarding to be able to help people become well!

"Let's give it two weeks, Lyn. Then we'll look at dropping the evening suppository."

* * * * * *

But Lyn called a week later. "Karen, my rheumatoid arthritis is starting to flare up. It's not bad, but I don't know what I'm doing wrong. I'm eating exactly as we have discussed. I haven't had any pain since we began, but now it's starting."

"Are you getting all your sleep?" was Karen's first question. This was the most important issue in arthritis.

"Well, not exactly. I've been extra busy at work."

Karen was firm. "Your sleep is of critical importance. Remember if you are extra busy at work, you'll require extra adrenalin to be able to meet those challenges. That means more work for the adrenal glands. If you don't compensate by the sleep that you are required to get, then the glands won't be able to come up with the corticosteroids that you need to keep you from the everyday frictional pain, much less the extra friction that will occur because you are doing more."

"But the busier I am at work, the less time I have for sleep," Lyn replied.

"Believe me, I understand the difficulty," Karen answered, "but if you want to keep arthritis from occurring, you'll have to keep a schedule that allows you the sleep. Keep in mind that you can catch up sleep."

"What do you mean?" Lyn asked.

"If it's not possible to get all the required ten hours in one particular day, then make it up during the rest of the week. Take a nap on Saturday and Sunday afternoons," Karen answered.

"But I've heard that a person can't make up sleep," Lyn said.

"You also heard that ulcerative colitis was incurable," Karen said. "We hear a lot of things, but it doesn't necessarily make them true. You *can* make up sleep. The proof will be in the doing. If you are behind on sleep, you will notice the rheumatoid arthritis raising its ugly head. Keep a log of the hours that you are behind in your sleep, catch them up, and you will see that the arthritic pain disappears as you catch up the sleep."

Lyn conceded. "Okay. I'll do it." She paused before going on. "Now for the really good news: I have had no blood in my stools for two months now, and I have totally quit the suppositories. I'm off all medications for my ulcerative colitis!"

"Absolutely excellent, Lyn! And the raw vegetables are going down all right?" Karen queried.

"Yes, I've even had tuna salad with raw celery and onions, and I had no problems."

"Good. Then we're almost there. We still have tomatoes, fruit, nuts, and seeds to go. Then you will be eating everything again."

"Except sweets," Lyn interjected. "When do they come back in?"

"Not yet," Karen answered, "and when they do they will be severely limited. Sweets are not good at any time for any one, so I will never agree to a daily dessert, but an occasional dessert will not tip the scales. But not yet, Lyn, not yet. Let's finish healing."

Lyn sighed. She really did love her sweets. Karen had said they were addictive, and she believed her. Why else would she spend so much time thinking about them?

* * * * * * *

The weeks went by and Lyn eventually added back all foods except milk, which Karen insisted should never return to her diet. She was even allowed one sweet per week. The bloody diarrhea never returned and ulcerative colitis faded from Lyn's memory just as a bad dream fades. Her rheumatoid arthritis never returned unless she neglected her sleep and then she would only feel some stiffness. The use of medications for arthritis was as distant a memory as the ulcerative colitis. The days when she had to crawl to the bathroom seemed ridiculously insane. Why had there been such a big deal made out of issues that were easy to correct?

* * * * * * *

Time passed. Lyn rarely talked to Karen anymore. There was no need. She remembered Karen telling her, "One of my greatest joys is to be able to say to a client, 'You don't need me anymore. You're well. Continue to eat well, and you will stay well.'"

13

CHAPTER 13

What Could Be More Embarrassing?

Jayne hurried to get the last file folder of the stack put away in the appropriate drawer. Now if she could just make it out of the room and down the hall a few paces before …a mild obscenity crossed her lips as she felt the familiar cramping and leakage.

Walking as normally as she could without appearing rushed, she desperately hoped she would not meet anyone in the hallway as she stopped by her cubicle to grab her "purse." She had purchased that bag as a disguise for a normal woman's handbag, hoping no one would comment on its size. She needed something to carry the extra clothes without anyone suspecting. The number of times that she needed those clothes were too many. One time was too many!

Alone in the small bathroom, Jayne felt a flash of anger. "Maybe I should just wear diapers! Then I wouldn't have to worry as much!" The problem was even if she did that, the smell would be a dead giveaway. She would still have to scurry to the bathroom to change.

"At least I have the advantage of not having to rinse things out in a public restroom," Jayne muttered to herself. "Well, not as public as some other restrooms." She flushed with embarrassment as she remembered the time when she was in a department store and didn't make it to the ladies room on time. No rinsing clothes in privacy in that bathroom!

Jayne wrung out the garments and stuffed them into a plastic grocery sack, then shoved them to the bottom of her bag. As she exited the little room, she pasted on a pleasant smile as if nothing was out of the norm. She dropped her little parcel off at her work station, making sure it was well-hidden, and continued down the corridor.

Jayne worked in a large medical facility as part of the administrative staff. Her job was to collect, deliver, and return files to the appropriate office or to the record room. In her rounds throughout the huge complex, she had memorized the location of every bathroom in the building, especially noting the unisex or one person johns. Some days, depending on what she ate the night before, she would stash her "purse" on the bottom shelf of the cart that she pushed from office to office. She never knew when the trouble would hit.

Her official diagnosis was irritable bowel syndrome. She had struggled with it for years, but in the recent past it had grown so unpredictable that she felt like a bag lady, always carrying spare clothes wherever she went.

Pushing away the thoughts of bowel leakage and the cramping that came with it, Jayne finished her rounds for the day. She had so much to do that she couldn't take a lot of time worrying about this inconvenience. Tonight, she was going to her daughter's house to celebrate the birthday of one of her grandchildren.

****

After Jayne finally got home, she fell into bed exhausted. "So much living to do," she grunted aloud. "I don't know if I have enough oomph to do all that living." Her energy levels fluctuated widely. Sometimes she felt enough get-up-and-go that she embarked with intensity on one of her crusades to help her four grown children. Then some days she felt she didn't even have enough strength to fight her way out of a wet paper bag. "Maybe everybody feels like this," she groaned as she turned over to try to find a comfortable position to sleep.

Jayne woke early even though it was Saturday. Even when she was tired, she didn't sleep well. Shrugging into her clothes, she managed to get some things done that morning before she had to get ready for her lunch date.

Jayne was looking forward to her meeting with her friend, Kim. They had known each other for years and occasionally they would carve out enough time to go shopping or grab a meal together. Jayne was meeting Kim at a restaurant in Eau Claire.

"I'm not sure if everything will work out with Tom," Jayne told Kim as they began their meal. Tom was the latest flame in her life. No, she didn't like that—he wasn't just another boyfriend, he was someone that she truly loved. *Or at least I think I love*, Jayne added to herself as her thoughts whirled.

Kim said, "Roger and I are doing well together. I hope that it does work out for you and Tom."

Jayne pushed the remaining bits of her salad around the edge of her plate. Sometime she was going to give a lot of thought to her relationship with Tom, but it was easier to go through each day without thinking too hard. If she spent too much time thinking, she might regret her two divorces and question what her real purpose in life was. Those were thoughts that were too heavy to contemplate right now. She would just cruise through each day taking them as they came.

As Kim was telling Jayne about her new interior decorating project, the grumbling in Jayne's intestines gave her forewarning.

"Kim, excuse me for just a minute. I need to visit the ladies room."

Jayne stood abruptly and made a beeline for the restrooms. She didn't pause to note Kim's raised eyebrows. She didn't have time.

Whoosh. She made it. Sweat had beaded on Jayne's brow despite the air conditioning. "What caused this crisis?" Jayne asked herself as she washed her hands and prepared to return to the table. "All I had last night at that party was a little bit of birthday cake. I even passed up the ice cream."

By the time she reached their table, the waitress had cleared away her salad dish. Maybe that had something to do with it, Jayne thought. Salad. But it couldn't be that. She had barely finished eating the last bite when the urge had hit her. It certainly couldn't cause trouble that fast.

As she settled in her chair, Kim asked, "Are you okay?"

"Sure. When a person has to go, they just have to go," was Jayne's simple explanation.

But Kim wasn't put off. They had been friends too long. "Jayne, I'm seeing a nutritionist next Saturday. Maybe you should come along with me."

A nutritionist! What in the world could a nutritionist do to help her with irritable bowel? She had heard over and over from the doctors at the clinic that diet had nothing to do with it. Jayne almost laughed aloud as she politely refused Kim's offer.

Kim tried from a different angle. "I want to lose some weight. That's why I'm going to see the nutritionist. Maybe we could work together and hold each other accountable."

"Now that might be something I would like to do," Jayne replied. She really did want to lose some weight. The scale kept showing higher and higher numbers every time she stepped on it.

It wasn't long before Kim had Jayne talked into visiting the nutritionist with her. Their purpose: to lose weight. It would be a fun project to work on together. They would e-mail each other every day to make sure that they were sticking to the diet plan.

"I'll contact the woman and make sure it's okay if you come along. She might want you to have a separate appointment, but I'll tell her we really want to be together," Kim said as they left the restaurant to go their separate ways.

"Sounds good. Just let me know," Jayne replied. Her spirits were lifted. She had enjoyed the lunch with Kim. The sun was shining and she still had the whole afternoon ahead of her to catch up with some of the home things.

* * * * * * *

"This darned throat of mine is forever acting up," Jayne complained to Kim as they drove to Fall Creek to meet with the nutritionist. "It's like I have a continual frog living there. I'm not sure if I have an on-going cold or a permanent sinus condition."

"Why don't you ask the nutritionist about it?" Kim suggested.

"She probably can't do anything for me. Remember, we're going to see this lady to help us lose weight. She probably won't even notice if I have a gravelly voice."

Kim shrugged. She really didn't know what to expect. It was actually Jayne's friend, Ashley, that had recommended this nutritionist to her, but she didn't know much about her except that any nutritionist should be able to help a person shed some pounds.

Fall Creek wasn't a long drive from Eau Claire and Jayne was glad. Unfortunately, she was going to have to use the restroom as soon as they arrived. Before even being seated in the woman's office, Jayne had to ask where the bathroom was. Kim was already ensconced in the small room that the nutritionist used for counseling by the time Jayne returned.

Karen Hurd was of an average height, slender, with dark brown hair. "It's a good thing she's not plump," Jayne thought to herself. "If she was, I think I would turn around and leave." Jayne had seen too many health professionals preaching the need to be the proper weight while they waddled around with twenty or more pounds padding their rear ends. Jayne reprimanded herself as these sour thoughts crossed through her head. What was the matter with her today? She felt out-of-sorts and grumpy. In fact, she felt almost like crying. Well, she certainly wasn't going to fall apart here!

The nutritionist started with Kim. Man! The woman was thorough. She asked every question that must have been in the book. By the time she was finished with Kim, Jayne was actually looking forward to her turn. Watching Karen deal with Kim was like watching a Humpty Dumpty production. Karen had picked Kim apart and put her all back together again.

Jayne did feel a little uncomfortable because the woman was so observant. Certainly, Karen wouldn't have missed the fact that Jayne had to visit the bathroom two more times while she had been talking with Kim. Oh well, everything was about to be laid bare anyway.

"Kim, if you don't have any more questions, I'm going to turn my attention to Jayne," Karen said.

"I don't have any questions now, but I might as time goes on," Kim replied.

"It's a lot of information."

Karen laughed. "You're right! You probably feel as if you asked for a drink of water and I turned on the fire hose. But I needed you to understand that there is a scientific basis for the things that I have asked you to do. Losing weight is not that difficult when you follow those five principles that I gave you."

Karen turned her clear brown eyes to study Jayne. In a soft voice that was full of compassion she said, "I think there might be a few more things with which I could help you than just losing weight, Jayne Halverson. In fact, I think weight loss is probably the least important issue that we should address today."

So began Jayne's session. As Jayne listed all the ills with which she had been dealing, she found herself relieved to finally be able to tell someone everything that she suffered. Yes, she had come here to find out how to lose weight, but she hadn't expected to find someone so knowledgeable in so many areas. Karen took notes in small, precise strokes that soon filled a page. When she finished answering all of Karen's questions, Karen laid down her pen and looked directly at Jayne.

"You've told me about the irritable bowel, the tendonitis in both wrists, the urinary frequency, the extreme fatigue, bursitis in your left hip, mood swings, hot flashes, lack of a gall bladder, and the anxiety. What you didn't mention are things that you probably haven't paid much attention to, but they speak volumes to me."

Jayne hesitated. What had Karen seen that she hadn't already told her? She didn't have to wait long to find out.

Karen said, "Your voice is quite raspy and you wheeze. And you have a persistent cough."

Good grief! The lady must have ears that could hear anything. Of course, Karen would notice the cough because she had been coughing off and on the whole time they had been there. But Jayne had forgotten about her gravelly voice. And she really didn't think it was that noticeable—no one had ever really mentioned it to her before—it was just the way she talked. She had had that sound in her voice for years. And as far as the wheeze, it was so slight and had been with her so long that Jayne herself rarely noticed it anymore.

Karen continued. "We may have some sinus drainage that is creating these problems; it may be some minor inflammation of the bronchial tubes; or we may have GERD—or a combination of two or all three of those. And if it's GERD, which is my first suspicion, then that will have most likely created the wheeze as well as the rasp."

"GERD? What's that?" Jayne asked.

"It's an acronym that stands for Gastro-Esophageal Reflux Disease. Heartburn is a simpler term," Karen replied.

"I don't have any heartburn," Jayne said.

"But you did tell me that you had your gall bladder removed years ago. That's a clue that you could possibly have some issues with GERD. The irritable bowel is another clue."

Jayne asked, "What does my not having a gall bladder have to do with my voice being the way it is, *and* irritable bowel?"

"First of all, know that GERD is only one possibility for the cause of the gravelly voice, as well as the wheeze. It could also be the other things I mentioned—and if it is then the solution is vitamin C and garlic. However, I want to explore the possibility of it being caused by some reflux—whether you feel the burning in the esophagus or not. Oftentimes a person will have mucous production from the irritation of bile in the upper gastro-intestinal tract."

"Okay, you'll have to explain that one," Jayne said.

"Years ago, prior to your gall bladder being removed, your bile had become so foul that it created irritation wherever it went."

Karen continued to explain to Jayne how the gastro-intestinal system worked, the recycling of bile; and how thickened bile created sludge and even rolled into stones creating gall bladder disease.

Karen finally concluded by saying, "Even though your gall bladder is gone, that doesn't mean we solved the bile issue. In fact, we didn't. The evidence of that is the irritable bowel that you still experience. The nasty bile can also create excess mucous in the throat which can cause a cough, a raspy voice, or many other things which you don't currently experience. We tossed your gall bladder in the garbage, but we didn't solve the problem of irritable bowel. And we may have this side issue of the upper respiratory problems caused by the same foul bile."

"How can the bile go up into my throat?" Jayne asked. "You explained that it was released into the first part of the small intestine." Jayne put her hand just below her sternum to indicate the place that Karen had just shown her.

"The gastro-intestinal tract is one long tube. Right here . . ." Karen indicated a place on her torso, "there is a sphincter—a muscle that opens and closes like the aperture on a camera. It's called the cardiac sphincter. It's called that because of its location. It's close to your heart. But it has nothing to do with the heart; it's part of the gastro-intestinal system. It's the same reason we call acid reflux, 'heartburn.' It's the proximity to that vital organ that we refer to—not that it is the troubled part."

Jayne nodded. She did understand that heartburn was not a problem with the heart.

Karen continued, "The cardiac sphincter separates the esophagus from the stomach. Then the tube leading from the stomach which is here . . ." she indicated a place underneath her left breast, "is a straight shot into the duodenum." Now Karen placed a hand on her duodenum. "The tube is interrupted by the pyloric sphincter. That little muscle controls the emptying of the stomach into the duodenum—when the sphincter opens the contents of the stomach move into the duodenum, when it closes the contents of the stomach stay in the stomach.

"When these sphincters open, some of the bile that is in the duodenum can and does backwash into the stomach. When the sphincters snap shut it can create back pressure which forces any stray bile up into the esophagus and even the throat." Karen indicated the upper center of her chest. "This is where the esophageal opening is. If the noxious bile gets up here it will burn just like it burns lower down in the intestinal tract. I always say that it's like General Sherman marching through the South, burning and pillaging as he goes. But what you need to know is that the bile can also create mucous production *without* any burning sensation."

Karen stopped and grinned, "You do know your Civil War history, don't you?"

Jayne nodded. She did, and she understood the reference to the general of the Union forces that wreaked such havoc in the southern United States during that period of history. Karen's illustration was clear. Recycled bile was a serious threat.

Karen continued, "The foul bile can burn wherever it goes—up or down. If the burning bile goes up, it causes heartburn. If the burning bile goes down—and it certainly does that—it can cause irritable bowel—as well as a host of other gastro-intestinal maladies."

"So not having a gall bladder doesn't mean that I don't have bile," Jayne said.

"That's it," Karen replied. "You will always have bile. If you don't, you can't digest foods and you'd be one miserable pup." Karen laughed. "And that's an understatement! Bottom line is that you must have bile to live."

"And we want bile that is not polluted with crud," Jayne said.

"Yes," Karen said, "and you need to know just a little bit more about anatomy. The esophagus is a tube that travels all the way back up your throat. If bile backs up further into your throat it can cause other problems such as excessive saliva, a burning tongue, a metallic or bitter taste in the mouth, mouth ulcers, and possibly even create problems with asthma. If the nasty bile causes inflammation, we will end up with a production of mucous to flush the bile away and this mucous can aggravate the upper respiratory tract. That's why GERD is sometimes misdiagnosed as asthma."

"But I thought that asthma was associated with allergies," Jayne interrupted.

Karen answered, "It most certainly is, as well as being associated with other inflammatory problems, but it is also associated with GERD. Please understand that I am not saying that if a person has asthma, that they have GERD. It just becomes one of the possibilities of the cause of asthma."

"But you think that my wheeze and raspy voice may be caused by bile backwash?" Jayne asked.

"I think it's a real possibility and one that we should address. If that isn't the cause, and it's strictly allergies or another inflammatory response for some other reason, then we will address those also."

Karen continued, "There's something else that you didn't mention when going through your health history. You don't get enough sleep, do you?"

"How in the world do you know that?" Jayne asked incredulously. Really the woman was almost uncanny.

"Just a matter of simple deduction," Karen replied. "It's no mystery. You're wearing the signs of it on your face."

Jayne reached up and touched her face. She didn't have any wrinkles, yet!

"It's your eyes," Karen said as she smiled. "You have significant dark circles and 'bags' underneath them."

"Oh," Jayne shrugged. "I've always had those."

Karen replied, "I would venture to say that you have *not* always had those, but it's been so long since you haven't, you just don't remember. Coon eyes always sneak up on a person."

"Coon eyes?" Jayne repeated.

"That's what I call those deep shadows and sagging flesh," Karen answered. "Allergy puffiness under the eyes often mimics the sleepless look, but yours definitely have the not-enough-sleep characteristics."

"Oh," Jayne said faintly. "I guess I do only average four to five hours of sleep."

For the next hour and a half, Karen spelled out exactly why she was recommending the things she did on Jayne's "lists." As Jayne and Kim stood to leave that afternoon, Jayne felt hope in her heart like she had not felt for …well, a very long time.

"Jayne, I'd like to see you in two weeks. Kim, we'll wait a month before you check in again. Jayne has a few more urgent problems that will already be showing improvement in two weeks and I'll need to adjust her lists. But the weight loss issue with you, Kim, will be well underway in a month without any changes to your lists. I expect that you will lose somewhere between five and fifteen pounds this first month."

****

The two women climbed into Kim's car. "Well!" Kim said to Jayne as she raised her eyebrows. "I thought you were only going to find out how to shed some pounds, but you ended up sharing your whole life story!"

Jayne was not at all daunted by her friend's teasing. "Karen has a way of seeing to the bottom of the barrel, doesn't she?" Jayne felt almost exuberant. "Maybe I'll be able to conquer this irritable bowel. That alone will be worth anything."

Kim laughed. "We have a lot of beans to eat!"

"I'm going to eat them. I have nothing to lose—except this horrible irritable bowel—so I'm going to give it a shot," Jayne said.

****

The first two weeks passed quickly. During Jayne's next conversation with Karen she told her, "The beans have been a miracle. I just can't believe the difference with my bowels. I think I can say that I don't have irritable bowel anymore."

"Beans do work rapidly," Karen smiled as she replied, "and your other problems will also clear up as we continue."

* * * * * * *

Jayne stood up from the comfortable wingback chair where she had been seated in Karen's office. A small inlaid table separated her chair from Karen's. It had been almost three years that she had been meeting with this woman. She had long ago ceased needing the nutritional counseling, but she came on a regular basis at her own request to just be reminded of the things she needed to continue to do. The changes in her life had been remarkable. She no longer had irritable bowel syndrome. She no longer had the wheeze. Her raspy voice and hot flashes were under control. She no longer had the coon eyes as long as she was getting her sleep. Tendonitis, bursitis, moods swings, fatigue, and anxiety were all things of the past. She had changed in so many positive respects that she was literally a new woman.

Their session finished, Karen also stood. Jayne crossed to her and hugged her. "Thank you for all you've done for me."

14

CHAPTER 14

It's a Good Thing I'm Home Schooled

Heather left the light on in the bathroom as she exited. She went to find her mother. The blood had not gone away. Nobody ever wanted to show another person, even if it was her mother, what was deposited in a toilet, but Heather knew something was wrong. At first, she had thought it a fluke, but blood every day for three weeks wasn't a fluke.

Cynthia Dillard was in the kitchen finishing the breakfast preparations.

"Mom, could you come here?" Heather asked.

Cynthia looked up. The tone in Heather's voice communicated a strong message of worry. "What's the matter, Heather?"

"You just need to come and see."

Cynthia followed Heather to the bathroom. When she saw the bloody stool, fear shot through her heart. The worst possible conclusions came to mind.

"Heather, we will get you in to see a doctor right away."

Cynthia's hands shook as she dialed the number to the doctor's office. What had happened to her girl that would cause this type of problem?

"I need to make an appointment with the gastroenterologist for my daughter."

"How old is your daughter?"

"Fifteen."

The receptionist replied in a polite voice, "I'm sorry, ma'am, but we won't be able to see your daughter. We don't take anyone younger than sixteen."

Cynthia explained Heather's situation to the receptionist, practically begging her to accept Heather as a patient. The receptionist put Cynthia on hold, returning a few minutes later to say, "We'll make an exception. The doctor will see your daughter right away."

In short order, Heather had her initial appointment with the physician and was scheduled for a colonoscopy.

* * * * * * *

Texas in April was beautiful. The weather was still mild and spring was in full bloom. But as Cynthia and Heather walked back across the parking lot at the medical facility, neither one noticed the beauty of the landscape around them.

"Do you feel alright?" Cynthia asked Heather.

"Just wrung out, that's all." Heather responded in a voice devoid of emotion. She gratefully sank onto the car seat once her mother had the doors unlocked.

"Mom, what does 'abnormal mucosa and aphtha' mean?" Heather asked as she laid her head back against the rest. She really was tired.

That was the finding from the colonoscopy. But it was the words "ulcerative colitis" that had stuck with Cynthia. She answered her daughter in as cheerful manner as possible considering how glum she herself felt. "The doctor said it meant you had some sores inside your intestinal tract. The pills that you'll be taking should heal them."

The pharmacy wasn't too far out of the way, and Cynthia stopped there to pick up the prescription on their way home. Heather stayed in the car while Cynthia went in.

When Cynthia returned, Heather reached for the prescription. "Asacol," Heather read the small container that held the pills, "Take two three times a day."

* * * * * * *

As each day passed, Cynthia kept hoping that Heather would report that there was no blood that day. But each day, Heather would shake her head as she came out of the bathroom. She was still bleeding. The pills weren't working.

The smothering heat of July was at its apex when Heather had her next appointment with the gastroenterologist. As Heather answered the doctor's questions, she wrote rapidly in her file.

"We'll have to increase the amount of Asacol," she said, "because you are still having blood in your stools. Hopefully that will take care of the bleeding."

Swallowing three pills three times a day was really no more difficult than swallowing the two that she was already doing. Heather shrugged and looked at her mother.

Cynthia voiced the question that she had been thinking for some time. "Is there any alternative to the medication that might be helpful to Heather?"

"No, there's nothing," the doctor answered.

Cynthia was disappointed. She hated the idea of her daughter having to take medications, and now more of them. But what else could they do?

The summer finally relented its merciless heat and allowed the cool breezes of late fall and winter to soothe the scorched land. Cynthia loved living in Texas but the heat really was overbearing at times.

"Mom, do you think I'm anemic?" Heather asked one morning. She was tired and looked washed out.

"You weren't the last time they checked," Cynthia replied. "Your next appointment is in January. That's not too far away. We'll make sure to ask the doctor to check your iron again."

Time passed. Heather, for all intents and purposes, seemed well to everyone around her. She was able to get her schooling done, participate in the youth functions at church, and live a "normal" life. However, Heather didn't advertise that every bowel movement she had was laced with blood. She simply accepted her diminished energy levels as normal and did what she could.

* * * * * * *

"We need to add another medication," the doctor said. Cynthia and Heather were at their scheduled appointment. "The Asacol is not taking care of the problem."

On the way home, Heather said in a very quiet voice, "Mom, enemas every night don't sound like much fun."

Cynthia didn't respond right away. She felt like crying. Fifteen-year-olds should not have to live on pills and enemas! Certainly, somewhere, somehow, someone knew something that could help her daughter. She resolved to start some serious research on possible alternatives.

That night Cynthia stayed up late. She was searching the internet for some kind of information that might help Heather. The number of returns when she typed "ulcerative colitis" into the search engine was overwhelming. She sifted and sorted through dozens of sites then ran across one that was very intriguing. It was like no other site that she had visited. The woman that wrote the article on inflammatory bowel disease explained everything so clearly. She had a plan for healing that Cynthia decided there was no harm in trying. They needed to do *something*!

"Heather, I think we should try this 'White Diet' that I printed off the internet," Cynthia said the next morning.

Heather took the paper and read it silently. She was sitting at the breakfast table. She had almost finished her bowl of cereal, but added a little more milk. Her mother was always encouraging her to eat more. She really was on the thin side.

"Mom, this says that I can't have anything but water to drink," Heather said. "What about milk? Milk is so good for a person."

"I think we should try the diet just the way it is printed," Cynthia responded, "even if you can't have milk."

Heather nodded. She really is a compliant teenager, Cynthia thought. Maybe having to go through all the doctor's visits and poking and prodding softened one's attitude. But Heather had always been amenable. Now, her younger sister, Hannah, was a different matter altogether. Cynthia smiled. She loved all three of her girls, each one so different.

"Mom, you're smiling," Heather said. "You haven't smiled in a long time."

Cynthia realized that Heather was right. The burden of Heather's situation had been so great that she must have let slip her normally cheerful disposition.

"I'll try to smile more often, Heather," Cynthia said. "It'll be a good thing for the whole family."

"Mom, can I go off my medications if I do this diet?" Heather asked.

That spurred a long discussion between Cynthia, Heather, and Heather's dad, Steve. After discussing the pros and cons, they made a bold decision. They would take Heather off all her medications and give this White Diet a chance to prove itself on its own.

Heather didn't complain about the plain and boring food that was on the diet. She dutifully followed the recommendations to a tee. Cynthia watched and waited to see if there would be any effect.

Day one, day two, day three, day four. Cynthia tried not to hold her breath. Heather was still bleeding, but she had been bleeding for months and the medications had not stopped it. She would have to give this diet a little time. But day five arrived and new symptoms came with it. Cramping and diarrhea made an appearance for the first time.

"Let's go back to the recommendations for day one," Cynthia suggested. "Maybe the diarrhea and cramps will stop."

Heather agreed. So back to day one they went. It was a blessed relief. The diarrhea and cramping abated. Day five arrived and again the diarrhea and cramping were back.

"I'm going to e-mail this nutritionist and ask for help," Cynthia said. That article had been written generically for a broad spectrum of the population. The woman even said in her article that each individual might need a variation of the plan, depending on their unique circumstances.

It was late that night when Cynthia got the e-mail off. She checked several times the next day for a response from the nutritionist. Nothing. She went to bed hoping that the lady would respond soon. Heather looked so wan.

The next morning Cynthia headed for the computer as soon as breakfast was over. There it was! A response from the nutritionist.

Dear Mrs. Dillard,

I do think that I can help your daughter. Living on Asacol and enemas is not the long-term answer. They are only treatments to relieve symptoms. We really need to look at the cause and correct that.

There is much that I need to explain to you, as well as things I need to ask you and your daughter. If you would like, we can set up a consultation. It will take about an hour and a half or so. If you are not local to Fall Creek, Wisconsin, we will conduct the consultation over the phone. If you are interested, you may call my office at 715-877-3510 to set up an appointment or e-mail me back.

Be encouraged. There are good answers.

Sincerely,
Karen R. Hurd
Nutritionist

Cynthia wasted no time in setting up an appointment. Heather had already lost ten pounds and the cramping had not abated. Before the day was out they had a time scheduled for the coming Tuesday. "Heather, do you think you will be okay until then?" Cynthia asked.

"I've made it this far. It's only diarrhea, cramping, and blood." Heather jokingly tried to make light of the situation.

Cynthia smiled. The girl really was a trooper.

* * * * * * *

"How many bowel movements a day are you having?" Karen asked Heather. The time for their appointment had arrived. Heather and both her parents were on the telephone to the nutritionist.

"Around seven to nine, but some days it's eleven," Heather responded.

"And do you have cramping?" Karen asked.

"Yes, but it's the blood that always worries me," Heather answered.

Karen was writing down every piece of information that Heather reported. "When you were on the Asacol, did you still have blood in your stools?"

"Yes," Heather replied.

"Karen," Cynthia interrupted, "she's had blood in her stools for eleven months now. The problems actually started about one month before we first saw a doctor. None of the treatments ever stopped the bleeding. They keep checking her for anemia, but so far there are no signs of it."

Karen asked many questions. Then she explained how the gastro-intestinal system worked, all about bile, and inflammation.

As Karen compiled Heather's "lists" she tapped her pen on the paper thoughtfully. She was listening to Heather's father, Steve, describe the atypical pattern of Heather's ulcerative colitis. Heather just didn't fit into the normal category of sufferers with ulcerative colitis. Most had cramping and pain accompany the bleeding. But Heather never did, until she went off her medication. It was possible that Heather had been seen by the doctor so early in the ulcerative colitis progression that the Asacol had really been effective after all. It had kept the cramping and pain from erupting, even if it hadn't stopped the bleeding.

"I think we need to do something that I normally don't ask my ulcerative colitis people to do," Karen said when Steve finished. "I'm going to add cod liver oil to Heather's list of things to do. Normally, I remove every bit of fat from the diet, but in Heather's case I think we are desperately in need of the anti-inflammatory qualities that the eicosapentaenoic acid in cod liver oil can give us."

"Eicosa...what?" Cynthia asked.

"It's a very beneficial omega three fatty acid that works at reducing inflammation by causing the release of healing thromboxanes. It's quite a long and detailed explanation, and I've probably overwhelmed you with enough explanations today, so suffice it to say that this fat might actually speed Heather's healing instead of slowing it as fats normally would."

"Omega three fats," Cynthia said. "I've heard of them before. That's what flax seed is known for."

"Yes," replied Karen, "but that's a different kind of omega three fat and won't benefit us in this situation at all. In fact, if Heather eats flax seeds right now, we will have major problems with increased cramping, diarrhea, and bleeding."

"Where does a person get cod liver oil?" Steve asked.

"It's normally found in health food stores, although some pharmacies and even grocery stores carry it," Karen answered. "But make sure that you purchase cod liver oil that has *not* been emulsified. The emulsified variety has quite a bit of sugar in it, and only one-third the amount of eicosapentaenoic acid that regular cod liver oil has."

It wasn't for much longer that Karen kept the Dillards on the phone. It had been almost two hours. Heather was tired. It was easy to hear that in her voice.

"I want to talk to you again in three days," Karen said. "By then we will have noticed some changes."

* * * * * * *

Heather faithfully did everything that Karen had recommended. The three days went by rapidly. She was still bleeding, but it was somewhat less.

"I had eleven bowel movements yesterday," Heather reported. "But the cramping is not as bad as it was."

"Is there any form to your stool?" Karen asked.

"No, it's all liquid," Heather replied.

"Karen, she's really tired even though she's sleeping well," Cynthia interjected.

"It's the white diet combined with the diarrhea that is making her weak," Karen replied. "We haven't seen much progress, but I'm not going to wait any longer to add back some of her proteins. That will make the difference in her energy level. I'd like her to eat the white meat of chicken at least three times daily, and as much as she would like to have of it. Otherwise, the diet is the same except that we need to increase the frequency of the cod liver oil to six times a day. And Heather, make sure that you drink that full half gallon of water. I don't want you to become dehydrated."

"Yes, ma'am," Heather responded.

* * * * * * *

"It's a good thing I'm home schooled," Heather said as Cynthia finished grading the paper that Heather had just completed. "Sitting with a heating pad on my stomach all day would be pretty difficult to accomplish in a public school."

Cynthia nodded. She was hoping that this diet would soon stop the cramping.

At the next scheduled appointment three days later, Heather reported,

"The cramping is even less than before, but I still lie on the couch with the heating pad on my belly for a good part of the day."

"There is quite a bit less blood in the stools now," Cynthia added. "It used to be when Heather was on the Asacol that the whole toilet would be red with the blood, but now there is only blood in the bits of mucous."

"Good, we're making progress," Karen said. "Now it's time for the soluble fiber. We add beans to your list, Heather. We're almost there. The cramps will abate very soon with the addition of the legumes."

"It hasn't been that bad," Heather said. Cynthia smiled to herself as she listened to her daughter on the extension phone. Heather had always had a high tolerance for pain and discomfort.

Cynthia said, "Karen, we've one more thing to report before we hang up. Heather's weight is down to 108 pounds. So it's only been two pounds that she lost since we first talked to you."

"You're doing a great job, Heather," Karen said. "You'll see that you will gain weight very soon and all this cramping and frequent bowel movements are going to slow down. We have the mighty bean that is entering the scene now!"

* * * * * * *

Three days passed. It was time for another consultation with Karen. Karen had wanted to talk to Heather every three days until Heather was out of crisis.

"The cramping is so little that I don't have to use the heating pad anymore. And my stools are becoming more formed—not so much liquid," Heather said.

Cynthia interjected, "Heather is like a different person. She is feeling so much better. And she has gained two pounds!"

After hearing the full report, Karen said, "I want to give the beans a little longer before we add anything else. Remember to eat your lean proteins, and don't touch a vegetable with a ten-foot pole. It's not time yet."

At the next appointment Karen could almost see Heather smiling across the phone lines as Heather informed her, "The cramping is gone. I'm only having one to three bowel movements a day and the stools are formed."

"And blood?" Karen asked.

"Only a drop or two in the mucous."

Karen nodded. Heather was coming along very nicely. They weren't there yet, but they were certainly making significant progress.

By the end of the first month that they had worked together, Heather was feeling great. She had gained weight, and although she still had some blood in her stools, the disabling diarrhea and cramping were under control. Her menstrual cycle caused a temporary blip on the screen of healing, but Heather bounced back after it was over.

Heather called in faithfully for her appointments that had spread out from every three days, to every week, and now every two weeks. Karen added different foods as the appropriate progress was made. By the end of three months, Heather was to the point that she was eating almost all foods again and had normal, formed bowel movements without any blood or even mucous. Only on the occasion would Heather see a trace of blood that came from the hemorrhoids that she had developed from the months of ulcerative colitis problems.

"Hemorrhoids take a little more time to heal," Karen had told Heather. Karen was still very strict with certain things in Heather's diet because as she said, "Until you are completely well without any symptoms, I will be stringent."

The weeks turned into months with no symptoms. By mid-July, just five months after they had begun, Karen told Heather, "It's time to set your maintenance diet."

"Maintenance diet?" Heather questioned.

"Yes, that's the diet that you should stay on for always. It's just good eating for anyone. You see, some things should never be a part of your diet, or anyone's diet, if you want to continue in good health."

"Things like what?" Heather asked.

"Like caffeine and artificial sweeteners," Karen answered. She went on to give Heather her "maintenance lists."

* * * * * * *

Time passed. Heather was no longer the sickly girl that spent her days in the bathroom or on the couch with a heating pad. She was robustly healthy with no ulcerative colitis.

Heather sat at her desk and finished composing the poem that had been on her heart and in her mind for months. Karen had once told her that she prayed for every client she had. She had said there was a window in her office that faced east, and she would go to that window lifting each one to God.

Dear Karen,

There is a person I want to thank
Who God has put in my life
And whose encouragement has lifted me up
So many times
I don't know what I would do
If she had chosen not to be used
By God
"You are special to me," she says
And I know it's true
Because she told me that . . .

She goes to her window of prayer
Lifting up to God the people in her life
Like clouds rising to the sky
Putting them in the hands
Of Him who reigns on high
Because she knows He's there
At her window of prayer

I am filled with gratitude so much

Every time I see
That I am learning to trust
And God is teaching me
Thank you for taking me under your wing
And for your discerning and caring heart
You have helped me find a new song to sing
And in my life you will always be a part.

For Karen, my nutritionist, who God has put in my life and who has blessed me so much, as a counselor and a friend.
Heather Dillard
Lubbock, Texas

* * * * * * *

Addendum: When I (Karen Hurd) e-mailed the above chapter in April 2006 to Heather and her parents to read for accuracy and approval prior to the publishing of this book, Heather asked if the following would be included in this chapter.

For the last three years, I've had to watch my diet, of course, to stay healthy. Since I am now in college, it has been hard to do and I must admit I have become somewhat more lenient with it. I still do have bleeding from the hemorrhoids. But I do feel better when I eat well, and I know that I need to continue in that in order to take care of my body. ~Heather Dillard

15

CHAPTER 15

Sometimes Life Is Like That

Brady pushed the mower a little faster. He had to finish all the trim work before dark. It was late August and the grounds-keeping work kept him busy. At least he didn't need the daylight to do the floor-cleaning jobs which would come later this evening.

No one would have known that the six foot, one hundred and fifty-four pound, seventeen-year-old had ulcerative colitis. Certainly he was thin, but he never slowed for one moment. He was noted for his staunch work ethic. His determination to accomplish his responsibilities in an excellent manner set him apart from his peers.

"Brady, you never complain," his mother commented as he came out of the bathroom after one of his many trips there.

"Why complain?" Brady answered in a matter-of-fact voice. "Sometimes life is like this."

Rhonda nodded. Brady was as pragmatic as she was. A person just dealt with whatever life handed out. It was as simple as that.

"Sit down for a moment," Rhonda said. "I want you to read an article." She waved her son over to the small desk that held their computer. "I found this on a web site today."

Brady shrugged but did what his mother asked. He had a great respect for his parents. They had labored long and hard to raise him. They had passed

153

on to him not only his work ethic, but the respect for human beings and their situations. Perhaps the pull that he felt to find a career that would involve helping people was because of his parents' values.

Brady sat down in front of the computer screen. Huh. A nutritionist from a nearby town had written the article. He read the lengthy piece. His mother didn't waste time watching him read but finished clearing and washing up the dishes from the evening meal. She had just as many things to do as Brady.

"Sounds okay," Brady said when he finished reading.

"So you're willing to try it?" Rhonda asked.

"Why not? I'm still having problems despite the medication the doctor prescribed," Brady answered. "What do I have to lose?"

The question was rhetorical. Rhonda knew her son well enough to see that. It was decided then. Brady would try this "White Diet."

But Rhonda wanted just a little more help for Brady than a generic article on a web site. "This nutritionist is in Fall Creek. Would you be willing to go see her?"

Brady thought for a moment. That meant spending money. He was like his parents in this way too—every penny mattered.

Rhonda knew exactly what Brady was thinking. "If it's too expensive I won't set up an appointment. Okay?"

"Okay," Brady agreed.

The next day dawned cool and breezy. But by noon it would be warm enough. Summers in Wisconsin were never blazingly hot, yet the temperature climbed high enough to make things uncomfortable at times. This day promised to be one of those hot ones. Brady gulped down his cereal and milk before taking off. He had a lot of work to get done today.

"Tomorrow morning I'm going to have the rice milk here for you," Rhonda commented as Brady was about to walk out the door. "What you had this morning was the last of the regular milk. I wonder if the store in town will have rice milk? If not, I'll drive to Eau Claire."

Bloomer was not that far from Eau Claire. In fact, many people who lived in Bloomer worked in the significantly larger town of Eau Claire. Rhonda liked living where they were in rural Wisconsin. There was no way she would ever want to live in a town as busy as Eau Claire.

As soon as Rhonda got to work and had a break, she placed a phone call to the nutritionist's office. She wanted to get Brady in right away. School started in just a few days. It would be a whole lot easier on Brady if he didn't have to visit the bathroom as often as he did now. Being at home or on the job was one thing. Having to leave in the middle of a class was another.

Rhonda hated having to spend any money, so she was grateful when she found that the cost of the consultation was very reasonable. But the reality was she would spend any amount necessary to get Brady well.

"We're set to see the nutritionist on September eighth," Rhonda told Brady when he came in for supper that night.

"Sounds good. Pass me some more of that bread, would you, Mom?"

Rhonda smiled. The kid was absolutely amazing. Despite the long day that he had put in, he still had a great attitude.

* * * * * * *

It was Thursday. Brady hurried to get his lawns done as soon as school was out. They were supposed to be at the nutritionist's office at 7:00 p.m. Brady was definitely willing to see this lady, even if it was only to acknowledge the help that she had been to him already. In the ten days that he had done the White Diet his diarrhea had stopped, and he had only one to two bowel movements a day versus the five or six that he had been having. Brady finished his work. He and his mother made it on time to the appointment, no problem.

"So you're a senior," Karen said. "What are you planning to do after you graduate?"

The nutritionist seemed interested in every part of Brady's life. Brady wasn't offended. He figured she needed to know some details so that she could help him in the best way possible.

"I'm planning on going to the tech college in Eau Claire. I'm interested in the fire fighter/paramedic program," Brady responded.

Karen nodded. It was obvious even from the short conversation that they had already had that this person knew what he wanted, knew how to get there, and had the determination to make it happen. Brady Bleskacek would be able to accomplish whatever he set his mind to. It was a privilege to meet such a quality young man.

The interview went on. "How many Asacol are you currently taking?" Karen asked.

"Twelve a day. When I was first diagnosed with ulcerative colitis they put me on three pills three times a day. But I still had the cramping, diarrhea, and some bleeding so they upped it to four pills three times a day."

"And did you improve with the higher dosage?" Karen asked as she wrote rapidly. She always recorded everything a client told her.

"No," was Brady's simple reply.

Rhonda filled in some of the details. "We found your article on the internet and began the White Diet. After just twenty-four hours Brady's diarrhea stopped. Since then he has had loose stools, but no diarrhea. Also, the frequency of bowel movements has decreased."

"This is good," Karen responded. "It shouldn't take us too long to see you completely recovered. The intestinal tract heals rapidly and we have youth on our side."

Rhonda looked the question so Karen answered it before Rhonda spoke, "The younger a person is the more rapidly they heal."

The consultation moved from questions for Brady to explanations of how ulcerative colitis can develop and what is necessary to cure it. Brady's only marked response, if one could call raised eyebrows a marked response, was when Karen told him that sweets would be a part of his "No List." Besides that, Brady listened with little reaction. He was fully attuned to everything Karen said, but he took the changes he would have to make in his diet as calmly as a stone takes the beating of the weather.

"Are you willing to do these things?" Karen asked Brady when she concluded.

Brady's response was typical for the young man that Karen would come to know better through the months ahead. "Yep."

So began the process of adding foods back in while slowly weaning from the Asacol. Karen talked to Brady on a frequent basis. It was late September by the time Brady was down to two Asacol a day, and he had gained three pounds. Everything went very smoothly, although Karen increased Brady's servings of legumes to six times a day rather than the three times a day, because she was not satisfied with the loose consistency of his stools. They needed to be formed and not like fresh cow pies.

"You've come as close to complaining as ever I've seen," Rhonda told Brady one evening as he pushed navy beans around on his plate.

"It's the beans. They get old after a while. But I'll stick to them," Brady said.

Soon the Asacol was no longer existent in Brady's life. He was eating venison hot dogs, peanut butter, cooked vegetables and, thankfully, fewer beans. He only had to eat those buggers three times a day now. And the best part was that he had no symptoms of ulcerative colitis—none at all.

But after almost two months of being symptom-free, Brady tried some highly seasoned elk sausage. Additionally, he had been pushing himself and as a consequence had been shorting his required hours of sleep. Diarrhea and blood in the stool were back. Karen imposed strict limitations on his already controlled diet and the number of bean servings went to five per day versus the three. Within a few weeks the relapse was over and Brady had returned to the point where he had been before the elk sausage. No more diarrhea, no cramping, and no blood. Karen continued to add foods and blessedly, the beans were back down to three times a day.

"Brady, you came through the relapse with no Asacol," Rhonda commented.

"I'm not planning on going back to the Asacol," Brady said in his matter-of-fact way. "It's obvious that I can take care of this with food."

Brady began the last semester of his senior year in high school feeling very well. He was eating most things, had gained weight, and had had no ulcerative colitis symptoms for months.

"I'm still not satisfied with the stools not being formed the way they should be," Karen said to Brady as they talked during one of the follow-up consultations. "Being loose and almost formed is better than they used to be but not good enough for total healing. It is the soluble fiber that will correct this final indication that all is not perfectly the way we want it.

"We have two choices: we can allow more time for the current amount of beans to finish the healing, or we can speed the process by increasing the number of times each day that you eat them."

There was no hesitation as Brady announced his decision, "I'll wait and give this amount of beans a longer time to finish the healing process."

Karen was not surprised at Brady's desire to leave the beans at three servings a day. She had learned early that legumes were not one of Brady's favorite foods. He ate them dutifully, but that was all.

Spring came on the calendar, but in Wisconsin it looked as if winter was still lingering. The piles of snow were melted to the point of just being patches in the shady areas, but the air was still chilly.

"I decided to do something," Brady told Karen in his typical this-is-just-the-way-it-is manner. "I went off the beans."

Karen waited because it was obvious that Brady was not done with his report.

"I was tired of them. I was doing so well, I figured I would see what would happen without them." Then Brady laughed. "But, I'm back on them now. It wasn't long before I was getting symptoms again."

Karen thought about the American diet. It was so woefully inadequate in soluble fiber—and in most people's diets, non-existent. Living without soluble fiber was as detrimental to a person's health as living without proteins. It wasn't as if the beans were acting as a medicine like Asacol; they were just essential to the normal healthy function of the digestive tract.

"Brady, beans are going to have to be a part of your life forever," Karen said. "They need to be a part of *everyone's* life if they want to have good gastro-intestinal health."

"I see that," Brady said.

"But it won't always be that you have to eat three servings a day," Karen added. "Eventually you will only need to eat them once a day, but we will need to increase them when you are under more stress.

"And Brady, we can do a soluble fiber supplement for those times when you are just fed up with the beans. Psyllium husk powder is soluble fiber and will accomplish all that the beans do."

Brady perked up. There was an alternative to beans? "How much of this psyllium stuff would I need to take?"

"Two teaspoons of the powder is equal to one serving of the beans," Karen answered.

Karen had just handed Brady a valuable tool. Rarely had Karen seen Brady display much emotion, but she heard a touch of it in his voice now.

"I think I'll try some of this powder," Brady replied.

The psyllium husk powder ended up working just as well as the beans. Brady was well. He graduated from high school and continued his education at the technical college. Lean, strong, and healthy, Brady was living the life that he was born to live without the crippling influence of ulcerative colitis.

16

CHAPTER 16

He's Just Not the Same Kid Anymore

"He's always grouchy," Greg's youngest sibling complained to their mother. "I don't even like to be around him anymore."

Phyllis tried to soothe over the complaints, "It's because he's not feeling well. Imagine how you would feel if you had all the problems that Greg does."

Phyllis was able to get everyone to go their separate ways. Too bad school was out for the year. It kept them apart from each other and the arguments were less. But her youngest was right; Greg really was irritable all the time. Well, they would see what the doctor had to say. Their appointment was scheduled for tomorrow. Phyllis was glad that the testing was complete. It had to be miserable to be poked so much and have all that junk shoved into you. Greg had tolerated it, but her heart had been torn watching him go through all those procedures.

"Significant Crohn's disease," the doctor announced as they sat in the small room. "The ileocecal valve is inflamed and the jejunum tissues are showing some changes. His C-reactive protein level is elevated and his liver enzymes are abnormally high."

Both Phyllis and Greg looked at the doctor blankly. The doctor said, "In plain English, it means Greg's small colon is irritated to the point of being sore and bleeding. The lab results just confirm it."

Phyllis was floored. It took her a minute to voice her next question. "So what do we do about it?"

"He'll have to go on medications," the doctor responded. "That'll stop the cramping, diarrhea, and bleeding."

"How long will he have to be on the medications?" Phyllis asked.

The doctor shrugged. "Probably the rest of his life. Treatment can help control the disease, but there is no cure."

Phyllis looked at Greg. He just sat there with an expressionless face. In the harsh lights of the office he looked even more ghastly pale than normal—or what at least had become normal for him. He hadn't always appeared so washed out. But it had been a long time since he had looked well.

The doctor continued. "Because Greg's ferritin and hemocrit are low, I'll have to put him on iron also."

"Is that because he's been bleeding so much?" Phyllis asked.

"Yes." replied the doctor. "We'll do regular checks on his iron levels as well as C-reactive protein and liver enzymes."

"What's a C-reactive protein?" Phyllis wanted to know as much as possible.

"It's a marker for inflammation. It is non-specific, which means it doesn't tell us where or what is inflamed—just that something is."

"And the liver enzymes?" Phyllis asked.

"When they are elevated it indicates that the liver is stressed and not functioning as optimally as it should," the doctor replied.

Phyllis felt the knot in her stomach grow. Sores in the intestines, low iron levels, and a liver that wasn't completely normal—besides the C-protein stuff. How could this be happening to her sixteen-year-old son?

* * * * * * *

"Mom, it's okay," Greg said. It had been several weeks since their appointment with the doctor. "I'm better. I don't have blood in my stools anymore, no diarrhea, and no cramping."

Phyllis sighed, "I know. But I don't like the idea of you having to take medicine all the time." Greg was taking two fifty-milligram tablets of mercaptopurine each evening. What she didn't say was that she had a gnawing fear that hadn't gone away ever since she read the insert that came with the prescription of the drug that Greg was taking. Those words were burned into her mind. "Mercaptopurine is a potent drug. It should not be used unless a diagnosis of acute lymphatic leukemia has been adequately established and the responsible physician is knowledgeable in assessing response to chemotherapy." When she had queried the doctor, he had said that the drug was commonly used to suppress the immune system. He explained that Greg's Crohn's disease was caused by his immune system attacking the small colon—so it was necessary to "quiet" the immune system. But it seemed so wrong that her son was taking a cancer drug.

Greg was continuing his defense. "It's working, Mom."

"Yes, but you still haven't gained any weight and you're as pale as a ghost," Phyllis responded. She shut her mouth. There was no sense in arguing. What could she or Greg or anybody do about the situation anyway? They were doing all that they could. Or were they? The thought crossed Phyllis' mind for the hundredth time.

The months went by. Greg was pasty pale and still painfully thin. He participated in life but there was no zest in his living. As Phyllis watched him on the basketball court during one of his games, she winced. Compared to the other boys he was scrawny and didn't move as fast. Greg had wanted to be involved in sports. He also played golf and lifted weights, depending on the season. Phyllis didn't discourage him in these activities. Everyone knew that exercise was always good for a person, but she worried because Greg never really seemed robust in any sense of the word. Their relatives even began commenting at family gatherings that Greg didn't seem very peppy and that he didn't look well.

Phyllis kept her ears and eyes open for any scrap of information that might help her son. Then by chance she learned of a nutritionist that didn't live too far away that had had success with Crohn's disease. They could make the drive from West Salem to Fall Creek.

"Greg, I'd like to take you to see this lady," Phyllis told him one morning. Greg shrugged. "I've set up an appointment for this Thursday."

"Whatever, Mom." Greg said. He finished his piece of cherry pastry and stood up from the table. A fit of coughing took him. He had been fighting a cold for days. "You think I should go even if I still have this cold?"

"Even more reason to go. You've been too sickly for too long." Phyllis knew that Greg wasn't resisting, he just wasn't very interested—in anything.

* * * * * * *

"So besides the Crohn's, you have a history of severe headaches, allergies, excessive sweating, and insomnia," Karen summarized.

Greg sighed. He really was tired. This cold had him down. He was glad that Mom was answering most of the lady's questions. He really didn't want to talk at all.

"And you've been on the mercaptopurine for how long?" Karen asked.

"Since he was diagnosed with the Crohn's. So over eight months now," Phyllis answered for Greg.

Karen did not let her sigh move her lips or shoulders. There was no sense in burdening these people. What we do in the name of health, she thought to herself. It is heart-breaking. Karen thought about all of her dear friends that were doctors. They were just doing what they thought was right. Isn't that what everybody did? What they thought was right? What is right?

Karen finished taking the detailed notes on Greg's situation. Then she explained what she felt was the cause of Greg's Crohn's disease. Phyllis listened closely. Karen even explained why Greg suffered with the excessive sweating, migraines, and insomnia. They were all linked to this adrenalin business which was directly linked to the Crohn's. "Adrenalin-laced bile" was how Karen explained the Crohn's. Even Greg's allergies were affected by this adrenalin process, at least indirectly. Phyllis could see the pieces fitting together: Greg's shy nature, the sweats, the headaches—and his diet! He had been eating all the wrong things. In fact, he had been eating things that would actually aggravate if not cause the Crohn's! Phyllis was completely absorbed in the woman's explanation. Karen had a way of teaching that made things easy to understand.

Greg sat listening, trying to take in as much as he could, considering how poorly he felt. The lady did seem to know what she was talking about. He would be willing to give the things she was recommending a try. What did it really matter? It was only food anyway.

* * * * * * *

"Greg, we'll have to wait on the corn chowder," Karen said a few weeks later. "It's still too early."

"Okay, just checking," Greg said.

"What is your weight today?" Karen asked.

"One hundred fifty-five pounds," Greg answered.

"Good, we haven't lost, but we haven't gained. We *will* gain though—in time." Karen added, "You do know that you are underweight for being six foot two inches?"

"Yeah, I know."

"Greg, you have been stable for so long—no cramping, no diarrhea, no blood, no constipation—we should consider a weaning from the mercaptopurine," Karen said.

Greg didn't respond. He wasn't so sure. His mom kept telling him what a bad drug it was, but he didn't want to go back to that bloody diarrhea business.

Karen sensed his hesitation. "Let's keep on with the diet. We'll see how you're feeling in a few more weeks."

It was the end of April, a little less than one month after their first meeting with Karen. Greg was calling in for his next follow-up appointment.

"Any headaches?" Karen asked.

"No," Greg answered.

"Are you sleeping any better?" she asked.

"Actually, I am," Greg responded. He hadn't really thought about that until Karen asked.

Karen continued through her list of questions. Greg's energy level was good and he had gained four pounds. Greg's diet was inclusive of almost all foods and he was in no distress.

Greg knew that he was feeling better. In fact, so much better that he was now willing to try the weaning from the mercaptopurine.

As the weeks went by, Greg continued to gain weight, his C-reactive protein levels went down, and he was completely off the mercaptopurine by the first part of June. It had been less than three months since he had started with the nutritionist.

"Mom, I don't even think that I have Crohn's disease anymore," Greg announced one morning as he finished eating his eggs and beans. "I can't believe how much energy I have."

Phyllis felt like shouting for joy. She had watched Greg change in the last few months. He wasn't that wan skeleton of a boy anymore. He was no longer anemic. The doctor said he could stop the iron supplements. He hadn't had any allergy problems or headaches; even the sweating at night was gone. He had gained over ten pounds and looked so healthy that people were commenting on it all the time.

"Greg, I want at least a year of no signs of Crohn's before I'll lower that bean requirement," Karen told him at one of his follow-up appointments. "We'll have to watch out for growth spurts because the increased hormonal production during those times can throw us for a loop—but the soluble fiber in those beans will keep any relapses at bay. Stay steady on those beans!"

"I'm solid on the diet," Greg responded. Karen smiled. It was so nice to hear the strength in this young man's voice. What a change from the first time she had met him.

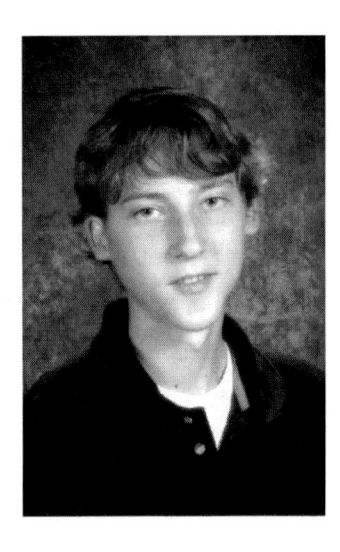

Greg Schneider, October 2004   *Greg Schneider, July 2005*

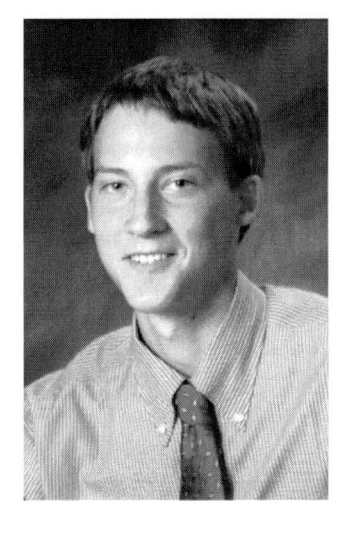

17

CHAPTER 17

Fingers That Stick and Feet That Burn

"All I can say is that my problems are really minor, at least compared to having cancer or heart disease, but they do irritate me. If I could do anything to make them better, I'd like to try." The woman's voice had a lyrical quality, its clarity only marred by the regular interruptions of a dry cough.

Springfield, Virginia, was a long way away from Fall Creek, Wisconsin, but Karen was accustomed to counseling clients via telephone. Through the years, she had learned that she could be just as effective using her listening skills as with her visual observations in discerning an unspoken problem. She did, however, always query her telephone clients on skin, hair, eyes, and body frame characteristics to fill in the gaps on areas she could not personally observe with her own eyes. Oftentimes, clients would send her pictures of themselves.

"How long have you had your cough?" Karen asked Mary.

"For three years," Mary replied.

"Three *years*?"

"Well, yes. Sometimes it gets better, but mostly it will be bad for two to three months at a time, then improve somewhat. Then it'll be worse again. It interferes with my sleep and drives me crazy.

"But at least the cough isn't painful. It's my feet and fingers that cause me so much agony. I've seen an orthopedic surgeon for my trigger thumb but didn't want to have the steroid injections or surgery. I went to a chiropractor for awhile but my thumb didn't really improve, so I tried acupuncture. That did help the pain, and the clicking in the thumb joint is better, but not totally gone. But now, my right ring finger is clicking and painful."

Karen finished taking Mary Bell's health history. Besides the cough, arthritic trigger thumb and finger, Mary suffered with eczema. She also described pain in her feet as so bad that it caused her to "limp like an old woman and I'm only sixty-three!"

Karen spent some time explaining to Mary the probable causes of her difficulties and the necessary solutions. Mary listened attentively. By the time an hour had passed, Mary felt like she was back in nursing school sitting in one of her most intense classes. But even with all the explanation, Mary still had a hard time understanding how her various health problems were related to each other. She knew her foot pain was caused by an injury to the fascia on the bottoms of her feet, her trigger fingers by a tendon problem. The eczema on her skin was a dermatology issue. Her cough—it was certainly a respiratory illness. She expressed all this to Karen.

"I know that they seem to be separate and unrelated issues, but for the most part, they are not. Your biggest culprit is the lack of corticosteroid production." Karen went on to emphasize the function of corticosteroids, their anti-inflammatory abilities, and how a reduction in inflammation could "cure" her fascitis, upper respiratory problem, and trigger fingers. Eczema was related to corticosteroid production but in a secondary fashion. Karen finished her explanations and gave Mary her "lists."

There was silence on the other end of the phone line when Karen concluded. Mary had long been interested in nutrition and was convinced that eating well was important for good health. But Karen was more than stringent! No sugar and no sweeteners would be the hardest rule to live with, but eating legumes every day was a close second.

"Mary, are you still there?"

"These are some lists! But as the medical doctors have had nothing to offer but steroids and pain medication, I'm willing to try it."

"Good for you!"

"Now, can I take garlic pills, or do I have to eat the raw garlic?" Mary asked.

Karen had told Mary the necessity of garlic for correcting her chronic cough. She had explained how it caused the mucous to thin and thus drain more easily.

"The freshly minced raw garlic is the most effective, and although there is some benefit in the pills, they don't have the power that raw garlic does," Karen replied.

"Okay, I'll do it," Mary said. "But this nine hours of sleep—I'm a very busy person and stay up late. Then, of course, I don't sleep well because of this nagging cough."

"Things will change and eventually it won't be so hard to sleep. The cough will clear up quickly and that will help us. But because you run on such large amounts of adrenalin, it will take us longer to completely conquer your insomnia. Remember that if you can't sleep the nine hours, you must *rest* the nine hours. And watching TV or reading a book doesn't count as rest. You may use those things to help you relax before going to bed, but they won't count toward your nine hours."

"Does the sleep or rest have to be consecutive?" Mary asked.

"No, just a total of nine hours for every twenty-four that pass."

When Mary finally hung up the phone, she took time to organize her notes. She would try to do all of the things that Karen recommended. If they would help her, it would be worth it.

That evening was a Creative Memories gathering that Mary was hosting at her house. The teaching of scrap booking skills was a love of Mary's life. She enjoyed this business immensely. Being a consultant for the Creative Memories company had become more than a job. It was a passion. The only thing that hindered her as she instructed people in the various ways to make an interesting portfolio was the handling of the small tools. Her arthritic trigger fingers would invariably get in the way.

As Mary made the preparations for the meeting her mind whirled. She would have to make a lot of changes in the way she ate. She grimaced as she spread the icing on the cake that she would be serving tonight. Things like this would have to go.

The meeting went well. Mary was in her element. Her enthusiasm covered up for the inability of her fingers to work the tiny scissors as effectively as she wished during her demonstration. Mary sighed with satisfaction, despite her creaky fingers, as she saw the last person out the door.

Mary cleaned the kitchen, tidied the living room, and prepared for bed. Oh yes, garlic. She was supposed to start that tonight. She squared her shoulders as she attempted to swallow the finely chopped garlic. But all her bravado did not help as the garlic came back up before it went all the way down.

"Okay, I'll put it in my food instead," Mary told herself with determination. But she didn't try it immediately. What she had just been through was enough for one night's experience.

Mary eventually found that a good quality garlic press made all the difference. She would put a small amount of plain yogurt in a tablespoon and put the raw garlic on top of it. Then she could get the garlic to slide down without even tasting it. Once she could take the garlic, Mary noticed an immediate improvement in her cough. Hopefully, the cod liver oil that Karen recommended for her eczema would work as quickly.

But as Mary climbed out of the pool two days later, she winced. Her eczema always flared when she went swimming. But she wasn't going to give up that sport despite her red raw flesh. Her entire family was involved in swimming. To take a Bell out of the pool was like taking a goldfish out of an aquarium. The results just wouldn't be pretty.

"I'll continue to grease up with creams and use the steroid ointment if it becomes absolutely unbearable," Mary told herself as she toweled off. "And what about that cod liver oil?" Mary mumbled. "I guess two days is really not enough time to see results."

Three weeks passed since her first consultation with Karen. By the time she had her first follow-up appointment, Mary was pleased to be able to report that her eczema had improved significantly after all. Her neck and chest had cleared so dramatically that she could honestly say that the eczema was almost gone. All she had left were the patches on the inside of her elbows.

"So I've done everything you have asked except for the nine-hour thing. I just can't stay in bed that long," Mary concluded.

Karen took extra time to reiterate the critical nature of obtaining the sleep. It was the crux of the arthritis issue. Mary agreed to try harder.

* * * * * * *

"I'm going to go," Mary said aloud. There was no one else in the room. Mary was arguing with herself. Former President Ronald Reagan had just died. The Lying-in-State in the rotunda on June 10, 2004, would be an event that she would always regret missing. But the pain in her feet had been so bad that to stand in line with the thousands of people that would be there would be a near impossibility. "I'll do it anyway." Her feet *had* improved some already. Maybe she could tolerate the pain.

* * * * * * *

The line moved slowly. Mary had been standing for over four hours and had several hours to go. But the magnitude of the event, the solemnity of the moment, and the high regard for this president kept her from leaving. The lights of the city of Washington, D.C. were a comforting backdrop as she waited her turn in the wee hours of the morning with the myriads of mourners who were also there to pay their respects.

As Mary filed by President Reagan's flag-draped bier, tears filled her eyes. A great man was gone. She was so engrossed with the event that she didn't even notice her feet. As Mary was driving home, the sun was rising over Washington, and a thought penetrated through the many others that crowded her mind. Her feet ached, but she had been able to stand for over eight hours. She had made it!

* * * * * * *

The months passed. Depending on the stress levels and the amount of sleep

Mary was able to get, the pain in her fingers waxed and waned. Her cough had cleared up completely. Her burning and aching feet were dramatically improved.

When George W. Bush was inaugurated in January of 2005, Mary spent the entire day in the nation's capital. She was able to enjoy everything from the Inaugural Ceremony to the parade, and then she went to the Inaugural Ball. Dancing at George Bush's Inaugural Ball was a dream come true. She realized that just eighteen months before, she would not have been physically able to do this.

* * * * * * *

"Now, ladies, let me show you a technique that will frame your pictures in such a way that . . ." Mary's voice modulated in her lyrical style as she continued her instruction. She was on her feet again, teaching at a Creative Memories activity. Her fingers worked the scissors with no pain or catching. Her feet didn't hurt. So many things had changed. Mary's health improvements added much enjoyment to her life. Eating differently, while challenging, was certainly worth every bit of effort it took.

18

CHAPTER 18

To Have More of a Social Life

Carol was seated in her living room. Practically everyone else was down in the common dining room. "But not me," Carol thought to herself. The residents gathered for meals, but the main draw wasn't the food; it was the fellowship.

St. James apartments were a facility for the elderly. Each resident had their own unit which included a kitchen, but meals were served for those who signed up for them. Of course, a person had to pay for them, but that was a minor point. The issue was that all of Carol's friends were down in that dining room visiting away, but she didn't have that option.

"My only choice is to be close enough to my bathroom so that I can make it there on time," Carol said aloud to herself. There was no possible way that she could walk or even run down the hallway to make it to her apartment in time if the urge came on her while she was in that dining room. There was a common bathroom closer to the dining room, but Carol knew she wouldn't even make it to that one. The urgency of the diarrhea when it struck was severe. If she didn't move very rapidly, it would be …well, bad.

"What am I complaining about?" she chided herself facetiously. "At least this irritable bowel is better than it was. Now I only have the diarrhea three times a day instead of nine times a day."

There was a buzz on the intercom system. Jean, her daughter, had arrived to take Carol to her scheduled doctor's appointment.

"Mom, are you ready to go?"

An ironic smile crossed Carol's lips. Ready to go. She was always going—but in another way.

* * * * * * *

The doctor listened to Carol's complaints about her intestinal issues, fibromyalgia, and other problems. She went over the medications and made adjustments as necessary. Carol really liked this doctor. She listened and seemed to really care.

"Carol, I'd like you to see a nutritionist about some of your problems. There is one in Fall Creek that I highly recommend. She is very knowledgeable and will be able to help you with this irritable bowel and fibromyalgia."

"I'm for that," Carol said. "I would very much like to be able to go places without having to worry about bowel accidents. And I sure would like to get rid of this pain."

The doctor wrote down the name and phone number of the nutritionist. Carol and Jean made their way out of the clinic.

"Do you want me to take you out to lunch before going back to the apartment?" Jean asked.

"I don't know if I dare," Carol sighed. She *would* like to go out to eat, but what if the urge hit her? It was too risky. "No, let's just go home."

Before Jean left her mother's apartment she said, "Mom, do you want me to call to set up an appointment with the nutritionist, or do you want to call?"

"You do the calling, Jean. You're the one that's going to have to drive me over there, so it's your schedule that we need to worry about. I have nothing going on." Carol waved her arm to indicate her small apartment. "And I'm not going to arrange any social engagements the way I'm feeling."

Carol lay propped up in bed that night, awake with the back pain that bothered her most of the time. She never could figure out what made it hurt so badly. The pain just seemed to have a mind of its own.

Her mind traveled back over the years that she had lived thus far. And it was a lot of years. Soon she would be eighty-six. She had lived a full and yes, at times, very stressful life. Those first few years when her husband had gone blind had been incredibly hard. For two years she was depressed. Then her mother died. Then her son died, the second child of hers that had passed on. She had never thought that she would be alive to see the death of two of her children. At times, the pain of losing her son was still fresh. Then her husband had died. Carol sighed. A long life was something that everyone always desired—including herself. But that meant that you had to see a lot of burying of people you loved dearly.

She listed off in her mind all the medical problems she had had through the years: ovarian tumor, appendectomy, hysterectomy, bladder tied up, gall bladder removed, Morton's neuroma, stenosis, mitral valve prolapse, back surgery, extensive cataracts, adrenal deficiency, diverticulitis, osteoporosis, spondylolysis, Hashimoto's thyroid, lichen planus, kidney infections, and oh, how could she forget? She wore hearing aids in both ears. And then the medications! How many did she take? Let's see, there was alprazolam, lorazepam, trazodone, allegra, synthroid, antacids, amoxicillin on and off, and . . .

She stopped thinking about it. She didn't tend to be morose. It must be the pain causing her to be so glum. Carol tried to shut her mind down. She really needed to sleep. She reached over to her bedside table and turned on the little tape player. The relaxation tape would help her to fall asleep. She turned off the lamp, and closed her eyes. But sleep only came for a short time. It wasn't long before Carol had to move to the recliner because of the back pain. She spent the rest of the night there.

The next morning there was a knock at her door. She suppressed a grunt as she stood to answer. The pain in her muscles was there again today, like most days. Carol opened the door to admit the smiling activities director for the facility.

"Carol, I have the month's menus for you. I know you haven't been joining us in the dining room, so you weren't there when these were handed out."

Carol took the proffered paper. "Thank you. But I don't think I'll be down for any meals for awhile." She really didn't want to tell the activities director why. It was embarrassing to talk about bowel habits. "But I'll keep the menu in case I change my mind."

Carol closed the door and glanced at the paper. The meals looked good. It would be so nice to walk down the hall and eat a prepared meal with the other residents. Carol took a few magnets and attached the paper to her refrigerator. "Maybe someday," she said softly.

Carol was looking forward to the appointment with the nutritionist. Today was the day, August 10. She was dressed and ready to go by the time Jean came to pick her up. They drove to the nutritionist's office in the nearby town of Fall Creek. The office had a pleasant setting. There were windows that lined three walls. The nutritionist had them open and the fresh Wisconsin air filled the room. Squirrels ran up and down a red maple just outside the window where Carol was seated in a beautiful wingback chair, and a woodpecker was hopping down the trunk of the horse chestnut tree that she could see out of the window near where Jean was seated.

Karen Hurd was a pleasant woman. And my, she could explain things. By the time the consultation was over, Carol felt like she had learned enough to fill a book. The recommendations that Karen made were reasonable, and best of all, it was just food. There were no pills that she would have to take—she took enough of those already. Karen said that she felt confident that the urgent diarrhea attacks would abate rapidly as soon as Carol started with the new eating plan.

Before leaving Karen's office, Carol arranged a follow-up appointment. Karen had said she wanted to see her in two weeks because the diarrhea would probably be cleared up by then and adjustments to her plan would be necessary. Carol felt like singing with the birds that were just outside those office windows. If the diarrhea was gone in a few weeks, she could have a social life!

Carol began Karen's recommendations immediately. "Who said an old dog couldn't learn new tricks?" Carol said to herself as she prepared her evening meal of efficient proteins and legumes. She opened the door of the freezer to get some ice cubes for her water and saw the half-empty carton of tofu dessert. "No need for this," she said as she tossed it into the garbage. She wouldn't be eating any sweets for a long time.

Everything went well. The diarrhea cleared up almost immediately. Carol was ready to try an evening out. She decided to accept her daughter's invitation to eat at a local restaurant.

Carol sat at the table studying the menu. "Why not?" she said to herself. She cleared her throat and told the waitress, "I'll have the deep-fried chicken and cabbage."

* * * * * * *

"I think the chicken was a mistake," she told Karen at their first follow-up consultation. "I've had no diarrhea except after that one meal."

"Any bloating?"

"I've had only a little. But it's nothing like it was before I came to see you," Carol replied. "And Karen, I haven't had any of those awful muscle spasms, and I've only experienced occasional fibromyalgia pain."

"Didn't you use to have that pain daily?"

"Almost daily. And I always took pain pills for it. But I haven't had to take any pain pills since I started coming to see you."

Karen finished taking Carol's report. Carol had more energy, she was sleeping better, "and last night I slept for nine hours straight. That's the first time I've done that in years!" Carol told her.

"You are a fast healer," Karen said.

"Doctors have always told me that, too."

"Well, you're holding true to your pattern. You're doing remarkably well for just two weeks. I expected the diarrhea to be gone, but the fibromyalgia and insomnia normally take longer to clear up. Carol, for being almost eighty-six years old, you're amazing!"

Karen added several things back to Carol's diet that she had to originally forbid because of the diarrhea. "We'll let a month go by before I see you again. By then we'll have even more positive changes."

* * * * * * *

Tomorrow was her next meeting with Karen. Carol lay in bed, not because she couldn't sleep, but because it was pleasant to lie there and think. "I feel so comfortable," she thought to herself. Carol pressed on her abdomen where she had had a tender place for so very long. It wasn't tender anymore. The diarrhea was non-existent. The fibromyalgia pain was almost one hundred precent gone, and she wasn't fatigued like she had been. She was off all her medications except for her synthroid. It had been five months since her first visit with Karen. She drifted off into a pleasant sleep.

The next morning, Carol was in her chair watching the morning news when there was a knock at the door. Carol easily rose without pain and crossed to admit the smiling activities director.

"Here are the next month's menus. It's been so nice to see you down in the dining room. I wasn't sure if you picked up a copy or not, so thought I would stop by with the listing."

Carol closed the door and sat down with a pen. She began to circle the meals that looked good to her. She would go down on Monday, Tuesday, Thursday—and oh—they were having meatloaf on Saturday! She would go down then, too. She caught herself humming as she finished marking the paper. She would be able to talk to Edna, show Florence the new pictures of her grandchildren, and finally tell Pearl all about the book she had finished reading. It felt so nice to have a social life again.

19

CHAPTER 19

But He's Just a Baby

Author's Note: The following chapter relates to one of my clients with liver disorders. I have included him in this book on inflammatory bowel disorders because the cause of many liver problems is the same as the cause of inflammatory bowel problems. The recycled bile that returns to the liver with its toxic components creates liver irritation and inflammation as readily as gut irritation. The answer is to not allow the bile to re-circulate. This is accomplished by the consumption of soluble fiber. The liver then heals because the cause has been corrected.

* * * * * * *

Liberty cradled her newborn in her arms. She was reluctant to allow the nurse to take him.

"It's only a little stick," the nurse tried to reassure her.

A little stick. Liberty winced. It was the repetition of the blood drawings that pained her. Her son was but a few days old and already he had had so many blood tests done that he was beginning to resemble a pin cushion.

"Maybe the test results will be better this time," Joshua said.

Liberty answered her husband in a worried voice, "I hope so."

It had all started when the hospital staff had noticed that Koleton was a little yellow. That was common, they said, but they would do a bilirubin count just to make sure everything was okay. But the test came back with high amounts of direct and indirect bilirubin in the blood. That's when the conferring with a larger hospital began. Something was wrong with Koleton's liver. They did all the tests again to make sure there hadn't been a mistake. But there was no error. For some reason Koleton's liver wasn't working the way it should.

"But he's nursing just fine. And he acts normal," Liberty told the physician as he was examining Koleton.

"I understand," the doctor replied. "However, the liver function tests are so abnormal that we must find out what is wrong. I have scheduled an ambulance to take him to the Marshfield hospital where they will be better able to care for him."

So from Medford to Marshfield they went. More blood tests. Each time the story was basically the same: abnormal. But Liberty and Joshua were hopeful because the bilirubin count was very slowly coming down although the medical professionals said it wasn't coming down fast enough.

"We'll put Koleton on soy formula and see if that helps. Maybe he isn't handling your breast milk well," the doctor said.

So they did that. But there was no change. Liberty went back to breast feeding her baby. And at least she had him at home now. They had to take him in for the lab work and doctor appointments, but he wasn't confined to the hospital anymore.

"I'd like to do a scan to see if there is a problem with the bile ducts," the doctor said. "And depending on what the scan indicates, we may need to do a liver biopsy."

"I don't understand how anything can be seriously wrong with Koleton," Liberty said. "He shows no signs of distress except for some fussiness before a bowel movement; he has gained two pounds; he nurses well; he . . ."

The doctor interrupted. "I understand, Mrs. Solberg. However, his direct bilirubin is 3.3, his AST is 103, his ALT is 73, and his total alkaline phosphate is 450. These numbers have not changed significantly since he was born three weeks ago. They are clearly indicative of hepatocellular dysfunction or infiltrative liver disease. I am scheduling the scan for March third."

So that was that. Liberty went home with her heart burdened. It didn't seem right. Were the doctors making a mountain out of a mole hill or was there truly something desperately wrong with Koleton? He was a happy baby. He was gaining weight. For all intents and purposes he appeared perfectly normal. The only thing Liberty could say that was negative was the way he was fussy before a bowel movement, but her daughter Olivia had been the same way. Wasn't it possible that the liver was just a little sluggish in getting going and that it would straighten out with a bit more time?

Each day that brought them closer to March third, the warning bells would again go off in Liberty's head. It just didn't seem right—a scan that involved radioactive dye and a possible liver biopsy! Everything in her heart rebelled against these diagnostic procedures. Her baby had already been poked and prodded enough. Joshua felt the same way that she did. But what could they do? Koleton's liver function *was* abnormal.

It was the evening of March second. Liberty was getting her young daughter Olivia ready for bed when the phone rang. It was her mother.

"Liberty, I saw a nutritionist today for the problems you know I've been having. But some of the things she talked to me about made me think that she might be able to help Koleton."

A flicker of hope sparked in Liberty's heart. "Did you tell this person about our situation?"

"I did. I didn't know all the numbers, but I gave her a rough outline of what has been happening. She said that she thought she could help Koleton."

"Mom, I want to talk to this lady right away. The scan is tomorrow."

"I know. I asked her if you could call yet tonight. She said yes, and gave me her home telephone number."

Liberty didn't waste any time. As soon as her mother hung up, she dialed the Fall Creek number.

...t at her dining room table listening attentively as Liberty described ...on's problem.

"I think it very possible that we can correct this situation with diet alone," she told Liberty. "Oftentimes the liver enzymes are elevated because of bile irritation to the liver tissue. That's probably the simplest way to put it, although there is a long and complicated explanation. The inability of the liver to clear the bilirubin is a clear indication of the bile re-circulation pattern."

"Can we come in to see you tomorrow?" Liberty asked.

"I'm booked back-to-back with clients tomorrow and don't have an opening until next week, but I'll tell you what to do tonight, and then when you come in to see me, I'll explain exactly why I have recommended the things that I will ask you to do."

"Koleton's scan is tomorrow morning. I don't want him to undergo it, neither do I want a liver biopsy," Liberty said.

"You won't be burning any bridges behind you if you decide to cancel the scan. If the things I ask you to do don't work, then you can always reschedule the scan and proceed down that path. However, if what we do is effective, the scan and liver biopsy will be totally unnecessary."

Karen continued, "Koleton is in no immediate danger. You've told me that he is healthy and thriving with no signs of distress except the fussiness with bowel movements. By the way, that little piece figures into this puzzle perfectly—and I'll explain that when I see you next week. But Koleton's liver is not going to fail in the next few days or even in the next few weeks or months. Although his enzymes are elevated, they are not *that* elevated. You have time to apply nutritional solutions."

"Tell me what to do and I'll begin it right away."

"Since you are nursing, I'd like you to express enough breast milk to dissolve a quarter teaspoon of psyllium husk powder. It won't take much. Feed this psyllium husk to Koleton each time he eats."

"He's nursing about eight times a day."

"That's fine. At each of those eight times, make sure he gets the quarter teaspoon of the psyllium husk powder. After he drinks that down, then you can nurse him as normal."

"Where can I find this powder?"

"They have it at the health food store in Eau Claire. They might have it in Medford. Metamucil is a brand name for psyllium husk powder. However, few places sell plain Metamucil. And it *must* be plain. It cannot be sweetened in any way—whether natural or artificial, and it can't have any flavors. Most stores sell Metamucil that is flavored and sweetened. That won't help us at all—in fact, it will hinder us. So it's plain psyllium husk powder that we're after."

Liberty found Joshua as soon as she hung up. She excitedly explained what Karen had told her.

"We have nothing to lose," Joshua said. "And Liberty, let's cancel the scan for tomorrow."

Liberty did find psyllium husks the next day, but not the powder. She put in a quick call to Karen to ask what they should do.

"Put it through a grinder and make it into powder. It'll crush easily enough," Karen said.

"Will a coffee grinder do?"

"Sure."

Liberty hung up the phone and pulled out the coffee grinder and cleaned it well. She didn't want a residue of coffee in this special bottle that she was preparing for Koleton. Karen was right. The psyllium husks turned to powder very nicely. She stirred one-quarter teaspoon of the powder into the milk that she had expressed. It made the milk a little thicker, and Joshua had to cut a slightly bigger hole in the bottle nipple so it could go through. But Koleton took it readily. Good. One dose down.

days, Liberty was already noticing a difference. Koleton wasn't anymore when he had a bowel movement. And his stools had more form to them. They had always been runny before. He also was sleeping better.

The appointment with Karen came. She took a history of not only Koleton's short five weeks since birth, but also a history of Liberty's pregnancy with him and a brief history of both her and Joshua.

"Interesting. You've had gallstones and you are only twenty-seven years old," Karen said to Joshua. "The apple doesn't fall far from the tree."

She explained many things that day, including a tendency in some people to have a higher hormonal production. "Hormones are cleared by the liver and placed in the bile. Higher than the average, yet still normal hormone production, results in a bile that is more aggravating. The clearing of the bile from the body becomes even more important in these genetically-prone individuals.

"As the vast majority of bile re-circulates to the liver, so do the bilirubin and the other waste products that the liver is trying to clear. The liver can become irritated which will result in higher elevations of the liver enzymes, as well as the bilirubin count being abnormal.

"Soluble fiber—which is the psyllium husk powder that Koleton is eating—causes the bile to be excreted from the body. The bile is tossed away in a bowel movement and does not recycle. Thus the aggravation to the liver is eliminated."

"We have another blood test scheduled for March sixteenth," Liberty said. "Will that be a long enough time to see a difference in his levels? That gives us only one and a half weeks that Koleton will have been on the fiber."

"Oh, yes. That's plenty of time. His levels should be down, if not totally normal by then. If they're not, then we can look deeper for other reasons that might be causing his problems. But, from everything that I have seen, he should recover with just the soluble fiber."

Liberty and Joshua were faithful to administer the psyllium husk powder with each feeding. March sixteenth came. At 11:00 a.m. Koleton's blood was drawn. They went home on pins and needles, waiting anxiously for the phone to ring. The doctor had said he would call with the results.

At 6:45 p.m. the phone rang. Liberty jumped to answer it. It was the doctor.

"Koleton's levels have come down. And his direct bilirubin is zero! There is absolutely no need for a scan, liver biopsy, or even further blood work. Your son is fine."

Liberty and Joshua were ecstatic. Before even calling the relatives to proclaim the good news, Liberty placed a call to Karen.

"It's working! He's okay!" Liberty gave all the numbers of the lab results to Karen.

Karen instructed Liberty on how much soluble fiber to continue. Koleton would need to take the psyllium husk in a reduced amount until he was old enough to consume the legumes that would take its place.

Before she hung up, Karen said, "'Let food be your medicine.' That's what Hippocrates said. What we put in our mouth has incredible healing power." Karen had tears in her eyes as she put down the phone. She took a moment to thank God for his healing hand in Koleton's life.

CHAPTER 20

Remove a Five-Year Old's Colon?

Time management. It was as simple as that. Karen had reworked her schedule so that she could accomplish more in the same amount of time. Funny, how a person wasted so much time worrying about things, and how little time it actually took to do the thing that the person spent two to ten times as much time worrying about. Stop worrying, start doing. Karen had decided that was one of the keys to making the most of the time that a person does have.

So finally, she had derived a method to keep up with the e-mails that she received on a daily basis. One more to go for tonight, then she would be able to shut down the computer and make it to bed on time. Karen was as strict on herself as far as the number of hours of sleep required as she was on her clients. In fact, she was as strict on herself as any client in any area—whether food, sleep, or lifestyle.

The text of the last e-mail read:

Dear Karen,

I have been reading your web site in regard to ulcerative colitis. The White Diet sounds intriguing; however, I am uncertain whether to try it. I should say I am uncertain whether to have my son try it. I have a five-year-old son who has been diagnosed with ulcerative colitis. We have been trying various medicines over the past year, all with minimal results. At this point, the doctor believes he would be better off without his colon and I am scared to death. My son weighs thirty-seven to thirty-eight pounds. I am concerned that trying the White Diet would be dangerous to his weight. He has not gained any weight in the last year. I am interested in trying anything that may keep him from the surgery alternative. Do you have any suggestions for me? Thank you very much for your response.

Sheila

No, NO, N O ! ! ! It was so wrong. Remove a five-year-old's colon! Tomfoolery in the extreme! Karen squeezed her eyes tightly shut and pressed her lips together. It was hard not to be angry. Sometime this all had to stop. How long would it take to change medical society so that this type of stuff wouldn't happen anymore? Fifty years? Seventy-five years?

Karen heaved a long sigh before typing the response. Allowing a surge of adrenalin because of frustration and anger would not help her or anyone. She, above all people, knew the damaging effects of too much adrenalin. Karen effectively stomped down the adrenal response and let her fingers calmly type the reply.

Dear Sheila,

I will say this as strongly as I can—it would be a grave mistake to allow your physician to remove your five-year-old's colon. Ulcerative colitis can be reversed and completely healed, despite your doctor's dire predictions.

I strongly urge you to set up a consultation with me. I need to work with your situation personally so that we can see total resolution and healing. Let me know if you would like to schedule a consultation. The initial consultation will last about one to one and a half hours. I will need to conduct follow-up consultations also. If you are not local to Fall Creek, Wisconsin, we will conduct the consultations over the phone.

Be encouraged. There are answers that are reasonable and that will work for your son's condition.

Sincerely,
Karen R. Hurd
Nutritionist

Karen hit the send button, shut down the computer, and turned out the lights in her office. It was definitely time for bed.

Karen slept well, as she always did. The alarm went off the next morning, and Karen rolled over to turn it off. She wouldn't rise immediately. She would take anywhere from ten to thirty minutes to wake up slowly. She purposely set her alarm earlier than the time she actually had to get up. Jumping out of bed only created an adrenalin rush. Karen vigilantly guarded against those superfluous wastes of adrenalin. She had more than enough things to accomplish each day and they needed adrenalin to be accomplished. She did her best to measure out carefully and allocate appropriately her resources of this precious hormone. She had more than the average person because of her wonderful state of health, but she would not squander her wealth.

Writing done. Breakfast eaten. Chores finished. Schooling completed. Now it was time for her nutritional practice. Ten-thirty a.m. and the first client of the day would call or come to her office. In any breaks between clients, Karen would accomplish a myriad of things on her "do" list, which included answering e-mails.

It was afternoon before Karen downloaded e-mails. The mother with the boy that had ulcerative colitis had already e-mailed back. She was anxious to begin as soon as possible. Karen gave the information to her secretary, Ruth, who called the lady to set up an appointment. It would be a telephone consultation. They lived in Colorado.

Four days later, Karen was on the phone with Sheila, the mother of Graeme.

"Graeme is having six to ten bowel movements daily," Sheila said. "He's on five milligrams of prednisone. He's also taking 500 milligrams of Asulfidine, once in the morning and again in the evening, and 1000 micrograms of folic acid."

"How long has he been on the Asulfidine?" Karen asked.

"Since June of 2003."

It was March 20, 2004. Almost a year. Karen shook her head. "And have you seen any differences in his bowel habits since then?"

"No. And we haven't seen any changes since he's been on the Imuran either. The doctor added that in November of last year. Before that he was on Remicade, but that didn't help either."

"So currently Graeme is taking prednisone, Asulfidine, folic acid, and Imuran?"

"That's correct. And oh, he takes Imodium at night before bed. He passes stool while he's sleeping and never even wakes up to realize it."

"And is there any blood in his stools?"

"No. It's the frequency and urgency that is the problem," Sheila answered. "The doctors said that his colon is so rigid that it doesn't have the ability to hold much."

Karen finished taking Graeme's history. He didn't have any other problems besides the ulcerative colitis. His energy level was normal, no sinus problems, no skin problems—only the gut problems.

"Does Graeme have a nervous or sensitive type of personality?"

"No. Well, at least he didn't used to be. He has always been a mellow kid until he started on the prednisone. Since then he's been wired."

Karen took the time to explain to Sheila what she believed were the causes of Graeme's problems and how they could correct it. Karen was very strict with Graeme's diet as well as recommending soluble fiber six times daily. She then arranged a follow-up consultation for four days later. There should be some signs of progress by then.

* * * * * * *

"I am so excited," Sheila said. "Graeme is beginning to have formed stools for the first time in years—in fact, since he was two years old!"

"Graeme is eating all his beans?" Karen asked.

"No," Sheila answered. "But we've been able to do the 'No List.' Graeme doesn't like the beans, so that hasn't been going so well."

Karen was pleased to hear that there was some progress, but she knew that Graeme would never completely heal without the soluble fiber. "The beans are the most critical piece in Graeme's entire healing plan," Karen replied. "We'll need to be creative in getting them down him. We can also use a soluble fiber supplement." Karen told Sheila about soluble fiber supplements—where and how to get them. "Begin him right away on this fiber. It's absolutely essential."

By the time one month had passed, Graeme was off all his medications and his bowel movements were under control, as long as he ate his beans or soluble fiber supplement.

"For being a laid-back little kid, he sure can put up a fight when it comes to eating beans," Sheila told Karen during one of their follow-up consultations. "But I'll be persistent. The supplement is really helpful."

Graeme continued to improve, gain weight, and was even able to attend Kindergarten which he hadn't been able to do in the past because of the bowel accidents.

"Karen, I am so very grateful. As long as Graeme takes his soluble fiber, he has formed stools and no accidents. He's eating all regular foods—except the few things that you said must always stay on his 'No List,' and he's off all his medications. The doctor is more than pleased. And there is no need to have any surgeries!"

APPENDIX

Recycling of bile, Footnote 1, Chapter 4
Enterohepatic recirculation is a process well-recognized by the scientific community. Bile is manufactured in the liver and deposited into the gastro-intestinal tract. Then the bile is absorbed in the terminal part of the ileum and returns to the bloodstream to be filtered by the liver. It is known that only five to ten percent of bile is excreted from the body while ninety to ninety-five percent returns to the liver via the portal circulation (1, 2, 15). The recycled bile is then re-secreted into the gastro-intestinal tract.

This fact has caused some consternation to the pharmaceutical industry in the development of medications that are primarily cleared by the liver (6, 7). Amphipathic and hydrophobic as well as high molecular weight substances are eliminated through the hepatic pathway (3). Enterohepatic recirculation has a direct affect on serum concentration of these substances.

Soluble fiber works in a similar manner as the pharmaceutical bile sequestrants, i.e. cholestyramine and ezetimibe (12, 13) without any of the negative side effects. The ability of soluble fiber to inhibit the enterohepatic recirculation results in an increase of the excretion of bile (1, 4, 5). The loss of returned bile acids to the liver upregulates bile acid synthesis (1).

The liver removes hormones from the bloodstream and places them into the bile fluids (9, 10, 11). This is substantiated by the considerable work that has been done by scientists for many decades (16). Hormones can be recovered from the bile fluids (8, 23). It is reasonable to hypothesize that the increase of hormonal production will result in an increase of hormone concentration in the bile. Bile that carries more hormonal messengers may have a direct affect on digestion as is indicated in the clinical symptomatology of patients who present with gastro-intestinal difficulties.

Corticosteriods reduce frictional damage, Footnote 2, Chapter 5
Adrenocorticoid hormones are secreted by the adrenal glands. One of their major purposes is to reduce inflammation (10). Stimulation of the production of glucocorticoids such as cortisol is accomplished by the adrenocorticotropic hormone (23). This hormone that is released from the hypothalamus to direct

the production of the anti-inflammatory cortisol also causes the production of beta-endorphins which reduce pain and create a euphoric effect. Therefore, a stimulus of the adrenocorticotropic hormone inhibits not only inflammation but pain. Virtually any type of stress can stimulate adrenocorticotropic production (23).

Adrenalin and vasoconstriction, Footnote 3, Chapter 5

The adrenal medullary hormones norepinephrine and epinephrine commonly known as adrenalin are known for their ability to cause widespread vasoconstriction resulting in increased resistance and therefore a raising of the arterial blood pressure (23). There are many causes for the stimulus of these adrenal medullary hormones including exercise, hypoglycemia, hemorrhage, and emotional stress (23).

Decaffeination process, Footnote 5, Chapter 8

The decaffeination process has undergone many changes since its inception. Originally the solvent trichloroethylene was used to remove as much caffeine as possible although total removal has never been possible with any method of decaffeination. In 1976, the National Cancer Institute tested trichloroethylene and found it to cause liver tumors in mice (17). Since the 1970's other solvents have been used for the decaffeination process. These solvents include methylene chloride (dichloromethane) and ethyl acetate. As methylene chloride is strongly suspected to be a cause of cancer in humans, many companies have ceased to use this substance in their decaffeination procedure (17). In the 1980's a process developed at the Max Planck Institute began to be adopted. This decaffeination procedure involves the use of supercritical carbon dioxide (18). Another technique uses water from the soaked beans which is then passed through carbon filters. This process is termed the Swiss water method. The flavor-charged water is then reused to remove the caffeine from the following batch of beans (19). The Swiss water method should not be confused with the indirect method of decaffeination using the solvent ethyl acetate to remove the caffeine from the water in which the coffee beans have been soaked. The ethyl acetate tainted water is then returned to the beans. This method is often called the "water process." Ethyl acetate is often labeled "natural" as it can be found in nature (21). Of all the methods used to decaffeinate coffee, the chemical solvent procedures are the most common (20, 22).

Eggs and cholesterol, Footnote 6, Chapter 10
Cholesterol is an essential part of life that is absolutely necessary for human survival. Cholesterol is present in all of the body tissues and without it normal function cannot happen (15). Studies of cholesterol intake associated with heart disease have been confounded as most studies fail to account for potential other features of the diet that raise blood cholesterol levels (24). Studies such as the Ireland-Boston Heart Study (25) and the on-going Framingham Heart Study (26) confirm that it is a combination of several dietary factors as well as other outside influences that can affect blood cholesterol.

REFERENCES

1. Huff, Murray. University of Western Ontario, Robarts Research Institute. 2005. http://www.biochem.uwo.ca/undergrad/385a/HuffNotesOct05.pdf.

2. The John Hopkins University. Pathology. "Anatomy and Physiology of the Gallbladder and Bile Ducts." 2005. http://pathology2.jhu.edu/gbbd/anatphys.cfm.

3. Vore, Mary. University of Kentucky. "Hepatic Recirculation, Phase III Elimination: Another Two-Edged Sword." 1998. http://www.ehponline.org/docs/1994/102-5/editorial.html.

4. Kritchevsky, D. (December 1978), Influence of dietary fiber on bile acid metabolism. *Lipids*, 13(12):982-5.

5. Eastwood, M., Kritchevsky, D. (2005). Dietary fiber: how did we get where we are? *Annu Rev Nutr*, 25:1-8.

6. Entero-hepatic Recycling – Methotrexate (1971). *JPS*, 60, 1128-33.

7. Pharmacokinetcs (including BBB Penetration). 2006. http://www.huntingtonproject.org/Portals/0/TUDAC.pdf.

8. Koechlin, Bernard, Kritchevsy, Theodore, Gallagher, T.F. (1949). Preparation of Deuterium Steroid Hormones from Bile Acids. New York: Sloan-Kettering Institute for Cancer Research.

9. Western Illinois University. 2005. http://www.wiu.edu/users/mftkv/Chemistry102/steriods.html.

10. King, Michael W. Medical Biochemistry. Indiana University School of Medicine. 2006. http://web.indstate.edu/thcme/mwking/cholesterol.html.

11. Chase, Chevy. The Hormone Foundation. The Public Education Affiliate of the Endocrine Society. 2006. http://www.hormone.org/endo101/index.html.

12. Kahlon, T.S., Woodruff, C.L. (2003). In Vitro Binding of Bile Acids by Rice Bran, Oat Bran, Barley and B-Glucan Enriched Barley, Cereal Chemistry. Vol. 80, p. 260-263.

13. Baringhaus, K.H., Matter, H., Stegelin, S., Kramer, W. (December 1999). Substrate specificity of the ideal and hepatic Na/bile acid cotransporters. *Journal of Lipid Research*, Vol. 40, 2158-2168.

14. Brown, M.S., Goldstein, J.L. (October 1985). The Nobel Assembly at the Karolinska Institue, 1985 Nobel Prize in Physiology of Medicine.

15. Bowen, R. (1998). The Role of Bile Acids as Hormones. Colorado State University.

16. Baxter, J.D., Webb, P. (2006). Medical Biology: Bile Acids, Thyroid Hormone, and Obesity, *Nature*, 439:402.

17. Coffee Decaffeination Process and Cancer (1999). National Cancer Institute.

18. Decaffeination Process. 2006. www.kraft.com/100/innovations/decaf.html.

19. Decaffeination Processes. Colorado Coffee Exchange. 2006. www.Roasters2000.com,.

20. Monthly Caffeination Information. INeedCoffee. Digital Colony. 2006. www.ineedcoffee.com.

21. Schoenholt, Donald N. (2006). Addendum: The Decaffeination Process. Gillies Coffee Company.

22. DiPaolo, David (2005). The Decaffeination Process. The University of Texas Health Center.

23. Bowen, R. (1999). Pathophysiology of the Endocrine System. Colorado State University.

24. Kritchevsky, S.B., Kritchevsky, D. (October 2000). Egg consumption and cornonary heart disease: an epidemiology overview. *J Am Coll Nutr*, 19(5 Suppl):549S-555S.

25. Kushi, Lew, Stare, Ellison, Lozy, Bourke, et al. (1985, March 28). Diet and 20-year mortality from coronary heart disease. The Ireland-Boston Diet-Heart Study. *The New England Journal of Medicine*, Volume 312:811-818, Number 13.

26. The Framingham Heart Study, National Heart, Lung, and Blood Institute, 1995-2006, www.framingham.com.

ISBN 1412082129-9